Vital Signs for Nurses

An Introduction to Clinical Observations

Vital Signs for Nurses

An Introduction to Clinical Observations

Joyce Smith
Lecturer in Adult Nursing
School of Nursing and Midwifery
University of Salford, UK

Rachel Roberts
Matron
Calderdale and Huddersfield NHS Foundation Trust, UK

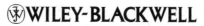

WILEY-BLACKWELL

A John Wiley & Sons, Ltd., Publication

This edition first published 2011 by Blackwell Publishing Ltd
© 2011 by Joyce Smith and Rachel Roberts

Blackwell Publishing was acquired by John Wiley & Sons in February 2007.
Blackwell's publishing program has been merged with Wiley's global Scientific,
Technical and Medical business to form Wiley-Blackwell.

Registered Office: John Wiley & Sons Ltd, The Atrium, Southern Gate, Chichester, West
Sussex, PO19 8SQ, UK

Editorial Offices: 9600 Garsington Road, Oxford OX4 2DQ, UK
The Atrium, Southern Gate, Chichester, West Sussex, PO19 8SQ, UK
2121 State Avenue, Ames, Iowa 50014-8300, USA

For details of our global editorial offices, for customer services, and for information
about how to apply for permission to reuse the copyright material in this book please
see our website at www.wiley.com/wiley-blackwell.

The right of the author to be identified as the author of this work has been asserted in
accordance with the UK Copyright, Designs and Patents Act 1988.

Library of Congress Cataloging-in-Publication Data

Vital signs for nurses : an introduction to clinical observations / Joyce Smith, Lecturer
in Adult Nursing, School of Nursing and Midwifery, University of Salford, UK,
Rachel Roberts, Matron, Calderdale and Huddersfield NHS Trust, UK.
    p. ; cm.
  Includes bibliographical references and index.
  ISBN 978-1-4051-9038-1 (paperback : alk. paper)
  1. Vital signs – Measurement. 2. Physical diagnosis. 3. Nursing. I. Roberts, Rachel,
1970- author, II. Title.
  [DNLM: 1. Physical Examination – nursing. 2. Vital Signs. WY 100.4]
  RT48.S 636 2011
  616.07'54 – dc22

                                                                    2010049555

A catalogue record for this book is available from the British Library.

This book is published in the following electronic formats: ePDF [9781444341867],
ePub [9781444341874], MobiPocket [9781444341881]

Set in 9/11 Palatino by Laserwords Private Limited, Chennai, India.

Printed and bound in Malaysia by Vivar Printing Sdn Bhd

1   2011

Contents

Contents

Preface

This book will provide a comprehensive resource for a cadet, student nurse or a registered nurse working within any adult healthcare environment. It is a valuable resource for registered nurses, allied health professionals or healthcare students undertaking or working towards a BTEC qualification, foundation degree or relevant in-house courses linked to vital signs monitoring.

Vital signs monitoring and the reporting of any clinical changes are fundamental in the delivery of quality patient care. Chapter 1 relates to legal and ethical principles and Chapter 2 reiterates the importance of infection prevention. Both chapters are integral to every aspect of healthcare delivery including vital signs monitoring. The remaining chapters focus on different aspects of physiological monitoring and a brief overview of the related anatomy and physiology. The concluding chapters discuss record keeping, reflective practice and continuing professional development. We hope this book will help healthcare professionals involved in monitoring a patient's vital signs link theory to practice, promote reflection upon their own practice and assist in their continuing professional development.

The aim of the book is to develop the underpinning knowledge and skills in both theory and practice for the adult patient found in hospital, private sector or community settings. This will enable staff to demonstrate their knowledge and skills when performing vital signs monitoring. In a changing National Health Service (NHS) climate, performing and monitoring vital signs, including good standards of record keeping, has never been more important.

Acknowledgements

We would like to acknowledge the Pennine Acute NHS Trust for allowing us to reproduce several charts and clinical procedures. Special thanks to the following people who kindly agreed to proofread chapters within the book:

Sylvia Maxfield, Infection Control Nurse, Pennine Acute Trust
Dr Tracy Birdsey, Lecturer in Diabetes and Physiology Open University
Lis Bourne, Lecturer in Health Care Ethics and Law, University of Salford

We would like to dedicate this book to our families for their support and patience as well as for accepting limited time together when the book took priority over many evenings and weekends. Special thanks therefore to Patrick, Eleanor, Irene, Marion, Robert, Emma, Helen, Ian, Matthew, Abbi and Eleanor.

Introduction

The focus on performing, recording and documenting vital signs has never been more important. For over a decade it has been recognised as problematic within clinical practice (McQuillan et al., 1998; Kenward et al., 2001; Goldhill et al., 1999; Goldhill, 2005). Research has highlighted that a patient's physiological deterioration has not been acted upon in a timely manner despite vital signs monitoring being an essential part of nursing care. In response to the concerns highlighted within publications by the National Confidential Enquiry into Patient Outcome and Death (NCEPOD) (NCEPOD, 2005) and the National Patient Safety Agency (NPSA) (NPSA, 2007a, 2007b), the National Institute for Health and Clinical Excellence (NICE) (NICE, 2007) has developed clinical guideline 50 *Acutely Ill Patients in Hospital and Response to Acute Illness in Adults in Hospital*.

In support of NICE clinical guideline 50, the Department of Health (DH) has reinforced the principles and standards set within the guidelines that NHS trusts must implement. One of the key recommendations states that anyone performing and monitoring the patients' vital signs be trained and assessed as competent (DH, 2007, 2009) as part of maintaining patient safety (NPSA, 2007a, 2007b).

This book is designed to be read as a whole or allow the reader to dip in and out of relevant areas of interest. The importance of each element of the patients' vital signs will be explored in more detail within each dedicated chapter. Within each chapter, learning objectives will be outlined to assist the readers in achieving their learning outcomes. The chapters will incorporate written and visual information for the readers to enhance their reflection during their learning experience. Case studies, activities or points for reflection have been included to relate the theory within each chapter to the reader's area of practice. Optional case studies and activity boxes are highlighted throughout the book as 'Practice points'. Taking the time to complete the practice point will encourage you to reflect on your practice as well as to evaluate your current knowledge.

It is hoped that this book will empower the readers to gain more confidence in their knowledge and skills in recognising and responding to the patient's vital signs. References and website addresses will be incorporated at the end of each chapter. At the back of the book is a glossary of terms that may be useful to the reader in explaining the **bold and italic** terminology used within the text. Answers to the practice points can be found at the conclusion of the book.

REFERENCES

Department of Health (2007). *Acutely Ill Patients in Hospital: Recognition of and Response to Acute Illness in Adults in Hospital.* NICE clinical guideline 50. London, NICE.

Department of Health (2009). *Competencies for Recognising and Responding to Acutely Ill Patients in Hospital.* http://www.dh.gov.uk/publications.

Goldhill DR, White SA, and Sumner A (1999). Physiological values and procedures in the 24 h before ICU admission from the ward. *Anaesthesia* **54**, 529–534.

Goldhill DR (2005). Preventing surgical deaths: critical care and intensive care outreach services in the postoperative period. *British Journal of Anaesthesia* **95**(1), 88–94.

Kenward G, Castle N, and Hodgetts T (2001). Time to put the R back in TPR. *Nursing Times* **97**(40), 32–33.

McQuillan P, Pilkington A, Allan A, et al. (1998). Confidential inquiry into quality of care before admission to intensive care. *British Medical Journal* **316**, 1853–1858.

National Confidential Enquiry into Patient Outcome and Death (NCEPOD) (2005). *An Acute Problem?* www.ncepod.org.uk

National Institute for Health and Clinical Excellence (NICE) (2007). *Acutely Ill Patients in Hospital: Recognition of and Response to Acute Illness in Adults in Hospital.* London, NICE.

National Patient Safety Agency (2007a). *Recognising and Responding Appropriately to Early Signs of Deterioration in Hospitalised Patients.* London, NPSA, Available at: http//tinyurl.com/yk8qbx5 [Accessed 26th March 2010].

National Patient Safety Agency (2007b). *Safer Care for the Acutely Ill Patient: Learning from Serious Incidents.* London, NPSA, Available at: http://www.nrls.npsa.nhs.uk/resources/?entryid45=59828 [Accessed 26th March 2010].

Legal and Ethical Principles

INTRODUCTION

Legal and ethical issues/dilemmas are abundant in healthcare practice and it is therefore important that nurses understand the law, ethical theory and professional guidance in order to be able to account for their practice. The law and ethical principles underpin all aspects of health care; therefore, as a member of the healthcare team, one needs to have an awareness of the legal and ethical issues that impact on healthcare professionals when undertaking and recording patients' vital signs. The legal, professional and ethical principles discussed throughout this chapter relate to adult patients only. All healthcare professionals taking responsibility for treating a patient thereby owe that patient a duty of care (Fullbrook, 2007a; NMC, 2008). The concept of 'duty of care' was introduced in Donoghue v Stevenson (1932) AC562 and Lord Atkin introduced the 'neighbour principle'.

> You must take reasonable care to avoid acts or omissions that you can reasonably foresee would be likely to injure your neighbour. Who then in law is my neighbour? The answer seems to be persons who are so closely and directly affected by my act that I ought reasonably to have them in contemplation as being so affected when I am directing my mind to the acts or omissions which are called in question
>
> (Dimond, 2008, p. 40).

LEARNING OUTCOMES

By the end of this chapter, you will be able to discuss the following:

❑ The legal system in England and Wales
❑ Ethical principles

Vital Signs for Nurses: An Introduction to Clinical Observations, First Edition.
Joyce Smith and Rachel Roberts.
© 2011 Joyce Smith and Rachel Roberts. Published 2011 by Blackwell Publishing Ltd.

- ❑ Professional regulation
- ❑ Consent
- ❑ Dignity and respect
- ❑ Equality and diversity

THE LEGAL SYSTEM IN ENGLAND AND WALES

The law, ethical principles and regulation by professional bodies underpin all aspects of health care. As a result of devolution in 1998, Scotland and Northern Ireland have their own healthcare legislation. The English and Welsh legal system is separated into three individual elements – the legislature, the executive and the judiciary. Legislation is the law passed by Parliament, which consists of the House of Commons, the House of Lords and the Sovereign (Queen). The laws made by the parliament cannot be changed by the executive or the judiciary. The executive consists of the police and local authorities; you may have read about cases that challenge local authorities when patients are unable to obtain the specialist drugs that they need. For example, women living in Wales who were diagnosed with early stages of breast cancer received Herceptin, but women in England had to pay for the drug because their primary care trust would not fund the treatment. Thus a 'post code lottery' that was dependent on which part of the country you lived in had consequences for women with early-stage breast cancer (Hendrick, 2004). The judiciary consists of judges who are independent from the government and parliament; however, they direct the interpretation of the law and must abide by the laws introduced by the parliament. All three systems work closely together to protect the public and ensure that the law is enforced (Boylan-Kemp, 2009).

There are two main sources of law that relate to England and Wales. They are Statute Law (Acts of Parliament), also European Law that is an integral part of the law in the United Kingdom, and Common Law (decisions made by judges based on previous cases) (Dimond, 2008, Montgomery 2003).

Statute Law (Acts of Parliament). The government, through the parliament, introduces a statute (Bill) or Act that is debated in both houses and approved by the sovereign. Examples of an Act passed by the parliament include the National Health Service

Act of (1946) that came into effect from the 5 July 1948, Data Protection Act (1998) and the Mental Capacity Act (2005).

Criminal law (criminal proceedings). These are usually brought by the state – for example in 1993, nurse Beverley Allitt was charged for murder and attempted murder on a children's ward; in January 2000, Dr. Harold Shipman, a general practitioner, was convicted on 15 counts of murder and the majority of his patients were aged over 65; and in 2008 Nurse Colin Norris was convicted of murdering four orthopaedic patients – all three were convicted in the Criminal Court (Ford, 2008).

Common law. Principles have been laid down by judges based on the doctrine of judicial precedent. Therefore, where a decision has been made, the principles of the decision shall be followed in later cases. In health care, a lawsuit regarding negligence will be judged under common law (Tingle and Cribb, 2007). For negligence to occur, the practitioner would have to deviate from a duty of care and so cause harm to the patient.

Civil law. A *civil action* is brought by an individual who sues another individual to obtain redress, usually in the form of damages and therefore may not be a crime. Any patient who is touched without their consent may pursue their action in the civil court as a tort of battery. The burden of proof in civil law is on the balance of probability with three conditions being satisfied. The first is that the practitioner was under a duty of care to the patient, a breach of that duty has occurred and as a result of this breach, harm has been caused to the patient (Pattinson, 2009).

ETHICAL PRINCIPLES

Throughout our lives, we not only abide by the law but we are also influenced by our morals, beliefs and attitudes. 'The word "ethics" comes from the Greek *ethos*, meaning character. "Morals" come from the Latin word *moralis*, meaning custom or manner – both words mean custom' and may be used interchangeably (Tschudin, 2003, p. 45). One definition suggests, 'Ethics is concerned with the study and practice of what is good and right for human being' (Thompson et al., 2000, p. 5).

Our morals may be influenced by our culture, religion or our upbringing. In health care, you may experience situations or decisions that you feel are morally right or wrong. Morals are based on our own beliefs and values; however, we have to respect that not everyone will have the same beliefs or values. To try to address the issues that may arise in health care, two philosophers, Beauchamp and Childress (2008), introduced a framework of four moral principles.

- **Respect for autonomy.** Respect for the right of individuals to make their own decisions according to their own values and goals. Therefore, we must respect our patients' rights to make their own decisions regarding any treatment or care.
- **Non-maleficence.** Obligation to do no harm. In all aspects of our care delivery, we must not intentionally cause our patients harm.
- **Beneficence.** Act in ways that promote the well-being of others. Always act in the best interest of our patients when delivering care.
- **Justice.** Treat others fairly. We must not be judgemental or discriminate our patients in relation to race, culture or disability. Every patient is treated equally with compassion, respect and dignity. Societal expectations are that everyone has an equal status in the allocation of healthcare resources. However, increasing costs and limited resources raise ethical issues and dilemmas related to health care.

In all aspects of our daily activities in practice, we may encounter ethical dilemmas when caring for our patients. An understanding of the law, ethical principles and professional regulation is necessary as it underpins our clinical decision making, including any actions taken. If you fail to deliver appropriate care for a patient, the legal and ethical principles are the same. Legally, if you are negligent you are responsible; ethically, you are also morally to blame for failing to take the necessary precautions to protect the patient when delivering care (Tingle and Cribb, 2007). In 2004–2005, there was more than '£500 million paid out by the NHS in clinical negligence claims' (Coombes, 2006, p. 18). As healthcare professionals, we have a legal, ethical and professional duty – not to cause harm to our patients who trust that we are competent practitioners (NMC, 2008).

PROFESSIONAL REGULATION

The Nursing and Midwifery Council (NMC) is responsible for the regulation of all registered nurses within the United Kingdom but ultimately its aim is to protect the public (NMC, 2008). To protect the public and ensure that registered nurses are fit to practise, the NMC has introduced mandatory policies, standards and professional guidelines for all registered nurses. *The Code* (2008) outlines the legal and ethical responsibilities and accountability of the registered nurse. If a registered nurse delegates to a member of the team who is not on the NMC register, he or she is held accountable for that delegation. Therefore, a registered nurse must ensure that the person to whom they delegate the task (e.g. taking and recording the patient's vital signs) has undertaken relevant training and been assessed as competent. The regulation of healthcare support workers has not yet been decided (DH, 2004). However, healthcare workers employed within primary and secondary trusts have been included within the Knowledge and Skills Framework and undergo mandatory training including the opportunity to access further education through National and Vocational Qualifications (NVQ) (RCN, 2007).

Equally, if the person undertaking the task fails to perform the task to the level at which they have been assessed as competent, then they are personally accountable in law (Storey, 2002). Consequently, the unqualified healthcare worker who delivers care to the patient is also responsible and accountable for his or her actions, while the registered nurse retains professional accountability. The NMC has a statutory obligation to regulate and monitor registered nurses and any complaints regarding a nurse's fitness to practise are investigated. The NMC Fitness to Practise Panel has the power to apply a caution order for 1–5 years, conditions of practice order for 1–3 years, suspension order for up to 1 year and to remove registered nurses from the register with no application to restore their registration before 5 years from when the order became effective (NMC, 2009).

Responsibility and accountability

Responsibility is a term that is used when you are responsible for your day-to-day actions and role responsibility is related to your contract of employment. It is important that you are aware of your responsibilities and accountability when you are delivering patient care. All healthcare professionals who are responsible for patients have a duty of care. A breach of duty is judged on whether an action or inaction has resulted in negligence. In Bolam v Friern Hospital Management Committee (1957) 1WLR 562, a doctor failed to inform a patient of all the risks associated with undergoing electroconvulsive therapy. The patient allegedly claimed that the doctor had not informed him of the risk of a fracture; also, he had not received relaxant drugs or been physically restrained during the procedure and therefore he stated that the doctor's management was negligent. Medical opinion was divided and there was no clear consensus on the treatment of patients undergoing electroconvulsive therapy. A decision was made by the judge to direct the jury 'that a doctor is not guilty of negligence if he has acted in accordance with a practice accepted as proper by a reasonable body of medical men skilled in that particular art'. The doctor was, therefore, not guilty of negligence as he had acted in accordance with accepted practice by the medical profession. The judgement indicates that a healthcare professional is judged on what is agreed as an acceptable level based on current practice, guidelines and policies.

All healthcare professionals are held accountable in both the criminal and civil courts and by their professional body. Therefore, healthcare professionals may be found guilty of a criminal offence against a patient in the same way as any member of the general public. If a healthcare professional is charged with gross negligence leading to a patient's death, they will be held accountable in a criminal court. For example, in Misra and Srivastava (2005) 1CRAPP R21, two senior house officers were charged with gross negligence and convicted of manslaughter over the mismanagement of a man aged 31 who died of toxic shock syndrome following a routine knee operation (McHale and Fox, 2007; Huxley-Binns, 2009) . The Court of Appeal held that the jury had been correctly directed that the negligent breach of duty had exposed the deceased to the risk of death. It was also highlighted during the court case that both doctors failed to recognise the significance of the patient's deteriorating vital signs.

As an employee, you have a contract of employment, and your employer is vicariously liable for your acts or omissions under common law. The legal principle of vicarious liability holds one person (the employer) liable for the actions of another (the employee) (Griffith and Tengnah, 2008). All healthcare professionals are therefore accountable to their employer and must abide by their contract of employment. If you do not practise within the employer's policies and guidelines, you will be held accountable for your actions. The employer is not legally liable if the employee has not adhered to their policies and clinical guidelines (Tingle and McHale, 2009).

Competence

How do you know that you are competent to perform a skill? To be considered in law as competent, you must have undertaken a training programme provided by your employer or higher education institution as part of your nurse training and been assessed as competent. Huxley-Binns (2009) cautions that nurses are at risk if they treat a patient and know that they have not been trained to carry out the treatment; this will result in a breach of their NMC 'Code'. In 1999, the government imposed a legal duty on NHS organisations to ensure that standards of quality patient care and best practice are evident within the trust (DH, 1999; DH, 2000). Clinical Governance was implemented to provide a framework within all acute NHS trusts to minimise risks and monitor clinical quality. In October 2008, the Department of Health carried out a national consultation on safeguarding adults from abuse and harm; 'Safeguarding Adults', a review of the 'No secrets' guidance was introduced in 2000. A key finding was that there was no adult safeguarding system in place within the NHS. From 2010 Safeguarding Adults is to be an integral part of Clinical Governance systems within the NHS (DH, 2010b).

An essential component of Clinical Governance is to ensure that policies, guidelines and training are available for all healthcare workers, thereby reiterating that education and training are integral in the development of a competent workforce. However, if following a training programme, you still feel you need further supervision and do not consider that you are competent, you have a legal and professional responsibility to inform the person who has delegated the task.

Practice point 1.1

It is a very busy morning on the ward and two members of the nursing team have telephoned the ward to say that they are sick. The staff nurse is trying to prepare for the consultant's ward round and telephones the on-call manager to request more staff. The staff nurse asks you to take blood from a patient who has just been admitted from outpatient's clinic. Although you have attended a venepuncture course, you have not completed the supervised number of blood samples that the Trust policy has stated you must complete to be signed off as competent.

Q1. What would you do in this situation?
Q2. Who is responsible and who is accountable for your actions?

Mental Capacity Act 2005

Within your area of practice, you may meet vulnerable adults who do not have the capacity to make their own decisions. Demographic studies predict that there will be 870 000 people with dementia by 2010 and this is expected to rise to 1.8 million by the year 2050 (Alzheimer's Society, 2006). Any patient who has been diagnosed with dementia may vary in his or her ability to consent to treatment. Patients who have had a cerebral vascular accident (CVA) or have suffered a traumatic brain injury may also be vulnerable. Patients may find it difficult to understand the information that you are providing and therefore unable to give informed consent. A lack of capacity to consent may be permanent or temporary – for example, a patient may be confused because of an infection or unconscious following surgery and therefore unable to consent (Nazarko, 2008). To protect vulnerable adults, the government has introduced the Mental Capacity Act (2005) for England and Wales that came into force in 2007. The aim of the Act is to ensure best practice, based on the principles of common law, and it consists of five key principles (Mental Capacity Act, 2005):

1. **A presumption of capacity.** Every adult has the right to make his or her own decisions and must be assumed to have the capacity to do so unless it is proved otherwise.

2. **Individuals being supported to make their own decisions.** Persons must be given all practicable help before anyone treats them as not being able to make their own decisions.
3. **Unwise decisions.** Just because individuals make what might be seen as an unwise decision, they should not be treated as lacking the capacity to make that decision.
4. **Best interests.** An act done or decision made under the Act for or on behalf of a person who lacks the capacity must be done in his or her best interests.
5. **Less restrictive option.** Anything done for or on behalf of a person who lacks the capacity should consider options that are less restrictive of his or her basic rights and freedoms if the options are as effective as the proposed option.

The Mental Capacity Act enables a patient to appoint another person who may be a relative, friend or colleague to be his or her lasting power of attorney (LPA) and have the power to act on his or her behalf in relation to care and treatment decisions (Dimond 2007c). The patient must have the mental capacity to set up the LPA, which only comes into effect once the patient no longer has the mental capacity to make his or her own decisions. A new development outlined in the Act is the office of Public Guardian that has been created to keep a register of LPA. Equally, if the patient has no relatives and does not have the mental capacity to make a decision in special situations, an advocate must be contacted. The special situations that apply include *serious medical treatment*, *accommodation arrangements by the NHS* and *accommodation arrangements by the local authorities*. NHS organisations and local authorities are required to appoint an Independent Mental Capacity Advocate (IMCA) to be available when special situations occur, to make decisions on behalf of those who do not have the mental capacity (Mental Capacity Act, 2005). The government has also produced a Code of Practice (DH, 2007) in line with the Mental Capacity Act that explains how to identify when a person is at risk of being deprived of his or her liberty. It is a legal duty to have due regard for the Code of Practice and any decisions by healthcare professionals regarding the patient's mental capacity and the appropriate steps involved in the decision-making process must be clearly documented in the patient's records.

CONSENT

It is a legal and ethical principle that valid consent must be obtained before treating, investigating or providing personal care for patients (DH, 2001). The Mental Capacity Act (2005) assumes that a person over 16 years of age has the capacity to make his or her own decisions regarding his or her care and treatment. For consent to be valid, it must be given by a patient who is mentally competent (Dimond, 2007a). There are three requirements for valid consent, that the patient has the capacity to consent, voluntarily consents and has the relevant information prior to consenting. Valid consent must be obtained without pressure or deception (DH, 2009). In Freeman v Home Office (1984), Mr Freeman was a prisoner who alleged that he had forcibly been given drugs against his will, thus claiming that he had not given valid consent because the prison medical officer administrating the drug had disciplinary authority over him and consequently he could not make a free choice. According to the law, the burden of proving absence of consent is on the claimant (patient). The Court of Appeal refused to accept his claim agreeing with the original verdict by the High Court judge: that the claim of coercion was rejected and ruled that the plaintiff had consented because he had been informed of the purpose of the treatment (Dimond, 2008; Pattinson, 2009).

According to the law, patients who are mentally competent have the right to refuse treatment. Equally, a patient must be able to decide to either consent or refuse treatment without pressure. To determine capacity, principles of common law provide legal direction – for example, in Re T (adult: refusal of medical treatment) (1993), T was rushed to hospital because of a road traffic accident, and following a discussion with her mother who was a Jehovah's Witness, T stated that she did not wish to have a blood transfusion. Following a Caesarean section, T was unconscious and haemorrhaged; although the medical profession felt they could not lawfully disregard her wishes, an appeal to the courts was initiated by her father and boyfriend. The court ruled that T should receive a blood transfusion (Whitcher, 2008; Pattinson, 2009). Lord Donaldson, the judge, noted that a special problem may arise if at the time of the decision the patient has been influenced by a close relationship. In his judgement, the patient's refusal was not therefore valid because of the influence of her mother. All healthcare professionals have a legal and ethical duty to respect patient autonomy; however, the cases presented highlight that consent may at times be a complex process (Dimond, 2007b, 2008; NMC, 2008). If a patient refuses the care you offer, the refusal must be clearly documented in the patient's care plan. The law also states that a person under mental health legislation is not necessarily unable to make a judgement in relation to his or her capacity to consent. In Re C [adult: refusal of treatment] (1994), a man in Broadmoor Hospital refused to have his gangrenous left leg removed. The doctors assumed that he was incapable of making a decision as he had been detained under the mental health legislation. However, the court took an alternative view as the judge was satisfied that he had passed a three-stage test – *firstly*, that he had comprehended and retained the information, *secondly*, believed the information and *thirdly*, made a clear decision after weighing his choices (Dimond, 2008). The law also states that the patient's previous wishes and feelings, if known, must also be taken into consideration including any written information. The patient's age, behaviour or appearance must not influence the decisions made in acting in the patient's best interest. The Department of Health (2009) recognises that partial consent may be given by the patient – for example, a patient may consent to a procedure but withdraw consent for certain aspects of that procedure. Therefore, a patient may give consent to undertake any tests that may confirm a diagnosis; however, he or she may, when advised of the treatment, decide to withhold consent to the treatment.

It is important that you gain the consent of the patient before you commence any procedures; an explanation of what you are going to do and the reasons must be discussed with the patient before you continue. There are several ways that a patient may give consent – patients may put consent in writing or consent verbally. Implied consent (non-verbal) may be expressed by visual observation of the patient's facial expressions or body language;

for example, this may involve the patient extending an arm for you to take their blood pressure or to provide a blood sample (Bourne, 2008; Dimond, 2008). The law recognises that consent for treatment can be in different formats and all are equally valid. However, the Department of Health (2005) recommends that consent for any major investigations should be in writing. This demonstrates that consent has been given and mitigates against a case of trespass.

Any procedure or any aspect of care that is delivered without consent has ethical and legal implications for healthcare professionals as patients have a right in law to take action in the civil court. Touching a patient without consent is called *trespass*, and *assault* is when the patient fears they will be touched against their wishes. Every patient who is mentally competent has a right in law to give consent to anyone touching his or her person (Dimond, 2007a, 2008).

Written consent is judged by the law to be the best and is the preferred method for patients who are having procedures undertaken that may carry any kind of risks – for example, prior to an operation. The Department of Health in 2001 has produced guidance on consent to examination and treatment that you can access from the website: www.doh.gov.uk.

Word of mouth is valid but may be more difficult to prove in a court of law and may result in one person's word against another. On a day-to-day basis, word of mouth will possibly be an important part of how you gain consent from the patient as part of his or her daily care.

Implied consent is when the patient does not verbally give consent. A patient may roll up the sleeve or put the arm out, ready for the blood pressure check and it is clear that the patient is giving consent to proceed (Bourne, 2008). Often, we care for patients who do not speak English and are from multicultural backgrounds. Therefore, it is very important that they are fully informed of any procedures in order to give consent. Several trusts now employ interpreters who translate for the patient; if there are no interpreters based at the trust, there is often a list of interpreters who can be telephoned to provide support for the patient and healthcare staff.

Practice point 1.2

Take time out to consider how a patient gives consent to any intervention or procedure. Make notes in the box below.

Consent	Verbal	Implied	Written
Vital signs			
Bed bath			
Venepuncture			
Medication			
Urine sample			
Operation/procedure			
Discuss treatment with a relative			
Discuss information over the telephone			

DIGNITY AND RESPECT

Every patient, especially one who is potentially vulnerable, has the right to be treated with respect and dignity (DH, 2001; NMC, 2008). Therefore, all healthcare professionals must treat patients with respect, dignity, listen to their concerns and act on their behalf. The Human Rights Act (HRA, 1998) clearly outlines under articles 3 and 14 respectively that no one shall be subjected to inhuman or degrading treatment or discrimination on the grounds of age, disability, race, gender, sexual orientation, religion or beliefs. In 2001, the Department of Health introduced the National Service Framework for Older People that emphasised that treating patients with dignity and respect was central to care delivery. At the same time, the government also established the Social Care Institute for Excellence (SCIE) that introduced a guide that respects people's dignity in health care.

The Dignity Challenge

High quality care services that respect people's dignity should:

1. Have a zero tolerance of all forms of abuse.
2. Support people with the same respect you would want for yourself or a member of your family.
3. Treat each person as an individual by offering a personalised service.
4. Enable people to maintain the maximum possible level of independence, choice and control.
5. Listen and support people to express their needs and wants.
6. Respect people's right to privacy.
7. Ensure people feel able to complain without fear of retribution.
8. Engage with family members and carers as care partners.
9. Assist people to maintain confidence and a positive self-esteem.
10. Act to alleviate people's loneliness and isolation.

(SCIE, 2008)

The Essence of Care benchmarks devised by the Modernisation Agency (2003) and updated in 2010 are benchmarks that compare and develop practice that is patient focused in line with best practice (DH, 2003a; DH, 2010a). Treating patients with dignity and respect is included as an essential benchmark. The Royal College of Nursing (RCN) initiated a national campaign for dignity in health care and advocated that all nurses should display respect, compassion and sensitivity; these represent the three characteristics of dignity when caring for patients (Waters, 2008). The NMC has provided guidance on patient dignity and care that relates to both hospital and community settings. Although the guidance is intended for nurses and midwives, the principles are applicable to anyone receiving health care irrespective of their age and should be utilised as a benchmark for principles of care delivery by all members of the multidisciplinary team (NMC, 2009).

Equality and diversity

On the 8 April 2010, the Equality Bill became the Equality Act (2010), addressing key areas in regard to socio-economic inequalities. The Act outlines seven protected characteristics that include age, disability, race, gender reassignment, religion or belief, sex or sexual orientation. All seven characteristics are integral to healthcare practice. Equality and diversity is an ethical principle of treating patients equally and respecting the diversity of their culture and beliefs. The NMC (2009) outlines equality and diversity principles as a personal commitment to provide care in a non-discriminatory, non-judgemental and respectful way. Equality is about valuing each individual and recognising that we all come from different cultures and backgrounds.

Practice point 1.3

John is 18 years old and has been admitted from the Accident and Emergency (A&E) department to your ward following a suspected drug overdose. The staff nurse from A&E informs you that they have contacted John's parents. You are taking John's blood pressure when he confides in you that he was at his cousin's party and has taken drugs, but that he does not wish his mum and dad to know. He asks you not to mention to his parents that he has taken drugs or that his cousin was involved when they visit.

Q1. What are your legal and professional obligations to John?
Q2. What ethical issues do you think may emerge from this situation?

Confidentiality

Confidentiality is a legal and ethical principle as the personal data of patients must remain confidential. However, there are exceptions to breach of confidentiality – for example, in W v Egdell (1990), Dr Egdell was instructed by solicitors representing a patient detained in a special hospital to provide a report for the patient's application to a mental health review tribunal. The doctor disagreed with the patient's resident medical officer and felt the patient represented a risk to the public. The patient's lawyers withdrew his report and it was not disclosed. However, Dr Egdell had grave concerns and made the report available for the hospital authority without the patient's consent. The patient's lawyers tried to restrain the report but the judge decided that the public interest in disclosure overrode the patient's right to confidentiality. The NMC 'Code' clearly states that you must only disclose information if you consider that someone may be at risk or harm and in accordance with the law (NMC, 2008).

As technology evolves and the number of patients requiring health care increases, there is a move away from the traditional method of paper case notes to electronic records. As a direct result of concerns regarding electronic data and maintaining patient confidentiality, the Government in 1997 appointed Dame Fiona Caldicott to review how confidential information is stored within the NHS. The Caldicott committee recommended the establishment of a network of Caldicott Guardians throughout the NHS. A senior person within the Health Organisation should be nominated as a Caldicott Guardian and the role was implemented in 1999 (DH, 1998; Fullbrook, 2007b). In 2003, following public consultation, the Department of Health (2003b) produced the NHS Code of Practice that relates to the consent and confidentiality of health records and includes the principles of the Caldicott report, the Data Protection Act and Human Rights Legislation. In 2006, the Department of Health published the 'Caldicott Guardian Manual'; the manual includes a set of principles and the fourth principle states that access to a patient's personal data should be on a strict need-to-know basis (DH, 2006). Confidentiality, therefore, comes under the umbrella of common law; there is a legal and also ethical obligation for everyone employed in health care to protect the patient's confidentiality (DH, 2003b).

CONCLUSION

In this chapter, the legal system that applies to England and Wales has been briefly discussed; thus it is important that you gain an understanding of the legal system in whichever country you practice (NMC, 2008). Ethical and professional issues related to patient care including the responsibility and accountability of healthcare workers in gaining the patient's consent have been identified as essential. It is also an important legal and professional requirement that you are competent in all aspects of the care you provide. Every patient has a legal and ethical right to be treated with respect and dignity including the right to refuse or consent to any procedure or treatment. Dimond (2008) succinctly states that nurses have a personal responsibility to stay updated on legal principles. An understanding of the legal, professional and ethical principles will therefore be invaluable throughout your career as the patient must always be at the centre of our decision making and care delivery.

REFERENCES

Alzhemier's Society (2006). *Alzheimer's Society Recommendations to Professor Mike Richards on a National End of Life Care Strategy for Adults.* www.alzheimers.org.uk [Accessed 23rd May 2009].

Beauchamp TL and Childress JF (2008). *Principles of Biomedical Ethics.* 6th edn. Oxford, Oxford University Press.

Bolam V Friern Hospital Management Committee (1957). 2 All E.R.118 at 122.

Bourne L (2008). Consent to treatment, patient autonomy and the law. *British Journal of Cardiac Nursing* **3**(9), 431–434.

Boylan-Kemp J (2009). The legal system. Part 2: it's not just for lawyers. *British Journal of Nursing* **18**(3), 178–180.

Coombes R (2006). Staying within the law. *Nursing Times* **102**(5), 18–19.

Data Protection Act (1998). www.hmso.gov.uk [Accessed 8th September 2009].

Department of Health (1998). *Implementing the Caldicott Report: consultation document.* www.dh.gov.uk/publications [Accessed 9th April 2010].

Department of Health (1999). *Caldicott Guardians.* London, DH (Health Service Circular: HSC 1999/012).

Department of Health (2000). *The NHS Plan: A Plan for Investment, A Plan for Reform.* London, The Stationery Office.

Department of Health (2001). *National Service Framework for Older People.* London, DH.

Department of Health (2003a). *Essence of Care: Patient-focused Benchmarks for Clinical Governance.* London, DH, NHS Modernisation Agency.

Department of Health (2003b). *Confidentiality: NHS Code of Practice.* London, DH.

Department of Health (2004). *Regulation of Health Care Staff in England and Wales.* A Consultation Document. London, DH.

Department of Health (2006). *The Caldicott Guardian Manual.* London, DH.

Department of Health (2007). *Deprivation of Liberty Safeguards Code of Practice to Supplement the Main Mental Capacity Act (2005) Code of Practice.* www.publicguardian.gov.uk [Accessed 12th March 2009].

Department of Health (2009). *Reference Guide to Consent for Examination or Treatment*, 2nd edn. www.dh.gov.uk/publications [Accessed 28th November 2009].

Department of Health (2010a). *Essence of Care 2010*. London, The Stationery Office.

Department of Health (2010b). *Guidance for Access to Health Records Requests.* http://www.dh.gov.uk/publications. [Accessed 6th April 2010].

Dimond B (2007a). Mental capacity and decision making: defining capacity. *British Journal of Nursing* **16**(18), 1138–1139.

Dimond B (2007b). The Mental Capacity Act 2005 and decision-making: best interests. *British Journal of Nursing* **16**(19), 1208–1210.

Dimond B (2007c). The Mental Capacity Act 2005: lasting power of attorney. *British Journal of Nursing* **16**(20), 1284–1285.

Dimond B (2008). *Legal Aspects of Nursing*. 5th edn. London, Pearson Education.

Donoghue (or McAlister) v Stevenson, (1932). All ER Rep 1; [1932] AC 562; House of Lords.

Freeman v Home Office (1984). 1036 AUER.

Ford S (2008). Could Colin Norris have been stopped? *Nursing Times* **104**(10), 8–9.

Fullbrook S (2007a). Consent: the issue of rights and responsibilities for the health worker. *British Journal of Nursing* **16**(5), 318–319.

Fullbrook S (2007b). Confidentiality. Part 3: Caldicott guardians and the control of data. *British Journal of Nursing* **16**(16), 1008–1009.

Griffith R and Tengnah C (2008). *Ethics Foundations in Nursing and Health Care*. Cheltenham, Nelson Thornes.

Hendrick J (2004). *Law and Ethics Foundations in Nursing and Health Care*, Wigens L. Cheltenham (Series ed.), Nelson Thornes.

Huxley-Binns R (2009). When is negligence a crime? *British Journal of Nursing* **18**(14), 892–893.

McHale JV (2009). Patient confidentiality and mental health. Part2: dilemmas of disclosure. *British Journal of Nursing* **18**(16), 996–997.

McHale J and Fox M (2007). *Health Care Law*. 2nd edn. London, Sweet and Maxwell Ltd.

Mental Capacity Act (2005). *Code of Practice (2007)*. London, The Stationary Office Limited. http://www.legislation.gov.uk/ukpg9/2005/9/pdfs/ukpg920050009 en.pdf.

Misra and Srivastava (2005). 1CRAPP R21, In: When is negligence a crime? Huxley-Binns *British Journal of Nursing* (2009) **18**(14), 892–893.

Montgomery J (2003). *Health Care Law*. 2nd edn. Oxford, Oxford University Press.

Nazarko L (2008). Choice, capacity, treatment and care. *British Journal of Healthcare Assistants* **2**(2), 82–84.

Nursing and Midwifery Council (2008). *The Code Standards of Conduct, Performance and Ethics for Nurses and Midwives*. London, NMC.

Nursing and Midwifery Council (2009). *Guidance For the Care of Older People*. London, NMC.

Pattinson SD (2009). *Medical Law and Ethics*. 2nd edn. London, Sweet and Maxwell.

Royal College Nursing Policy Unit (2007). *The Regulation of Health Care Support Workers*. Policy Briefing 11/2007. London, Royal College of Nursing.

Social Care Institute for Excellence (2008). *Adults' Services Practice Guide 9 Dignity in Care*. www.scie.org.uk

The Stationery Office (1998). *Human Rights Act 1998*. London, The Stationery Office.

Storey L (2002). Summary paper, presented by Les Storey, Senior Lecturer, University of Central Lancashire 4th Royal College of Nursing Joint Education Forums' Conference De Vere Hotel, Blackpool, United Kingdom. The 'Crackerjack' model of nursing and its relationship to accountability. *Nurse Education in Practice* **2**, 133–141.

Thompson IE, Melia KM and Boyd KM (2000). *Nursing Ethics*. 4th edn. Edinburgh, Churchill Livingstone.

Tingle J and Cribb A (2007). *Nursing Law and Ethics*. 3rd edn. Oxford, Blackwell Publishing Ltd.

Tingle J and McHale J (2009). Specialist healthcare law for nurses: an introduction. *British Journal of Nursing* **18**(1), 38–39.

Tschudin V (2003). *Ethics in Nursing: The Caring Relationship*. 3rd edn., Oxford, Butterworth Heinemann.

Waters A (2008). Dignity in action. *Nursing Standard* **23**(14), 17–22.

Whitcher J (2008). Legal responsibilities: consent in emergency treatment. *Nursing Standard* **23**(9), 35–42.

FURTHER READING

Office of Public Sector Information. www.opsi.gov.uk. [12th March 2009].

Infection Prevention

INTRODUCTION

On average, 800 people a day will develop a healthcare-acquired infection (HCAI) while in the care of the National Health Service (NHS). The Department of Health (DH, 2008, p. 1) Code of Practice defines an HCAI as:

> Any infection by any infectious agent acquired as a consequence of a person's treatment by the NHS or which is acquired by a health care worker in the course of their NHS duties. The prevention and control of HCAIs is a high priority for all parts of the NHS.

This means that at least 300,000 NHS patients per year develop an HCAI. A patient with an HCAI will stay in hospital longer and is more likely than uninfected patients to die. As the National Patient Safety Slogan goes, 'CLEAN HANDS SAVE LIVES' (National Patient Safety Agency, 2008). Patients, whatever their location, whether in hospital or within the community setting, need to feel and know that they are being safely cared for and treated and that healthcare workers are taking practical measures to reduce and prevent infection. Patients can easily lose their trust and confidence when observing poor practice in healthcare workers because of their fear of catching an infection. The nursing team is on the frontline dealing with patients and, in many cases, is a patient's first contact within the healthcare system. Therefore, nurses have a key part to play in *infection prevention* and it is an integral part of undertaking clinical observations.

Vital Signs for Nurses: An Introduction to Clinical Observations, First Edition.
Joyce Smith and Rachel Roberts.
© 2011 Joyce Smith and Rachel Roberts. Published 2011 by Blackwell Publishing Ltd.

LEARNING OUTCOMES

By the end of this chapter, you will be able to discuss the following:

- ❑ What micro-organisms are
- ❑ How micro-organisms spread
- ❑ The chain of infection
- ❑ How to break the chain of infection
- ❑ The four areas of Standard Principles (SP) for preventing HCAIs
- ❑ Responsibility for infection prevention

WHAT ARE MICRO-ORGANISMS?

'Micro' means small and 'organism' means a living individual consisting of a single cell or part of a group of interdependent parts (Oxford Dictionary, 2008). Micro-organisms cannot be visibly seen by our eyes and to observe them you would have to look through a microscope. Micro-organisms can also be referred to as microbes. Microbes or micro-organisms are invisible, tiny life forms that live in the world with humans. There are four main types of micro-organisms. These are bacteria, viruses, fungi and protozoa.

Many microbes are not harmful and in fact can live on and inside the human body. There are good micro-organisms (*commensal microbes*) that live in the human body as well as bad, disease causing micro-organisms (*pathogenic microbes*). Most micro-organisms are vital to human health and well-being. Micro-organisms will reproduce themselves in an environment that is warm with a temperature environment of 37°C, moist and damp. The human body, through the control of the immune system and the body's natural defences, prevents micro-organisms from causing harm. The body's natural defence mechanisms consist of the skin, the respiratory tract, the eyes, the kidney and the bladder as well as the digestive system.

The skin is the body's first line of defence. As long as the skin is intact with no breaks in it, it will prevent microbes from getting inside the body. When cells of the skin die, they fall off the body and accumulate in the environment as *dust;* they can live happily in a dusty environment for as long as 6 months. If there is a warm, moist and damp environment, the microbes in the dust will begin to reproduce themselves.

Sometimes, particles of micro-organisms can be inhaled into the respiratory system. However, within the respiratory system are hairs called cilia that waft the particles upwards and the body will get rid of them by making us cough or sneeze. The eyes will blink and also produce tears to help get rid of particles of micro-organisms.

Some micro-organisms invade the body in other ways and to prevent them from growing, the body has some natural chemicals to kill them off. For example, we have hydrochloric acid in our stomach, which will kill off any microbes that were ingested with food. Sometimes the body will make a person vomit in order to get rid of the harmful micro-organisms. The body also uses our senses to taste and smell micro-organisms. For example, tasting sour milk sends a message to the brain that it is unpleasant and potentially harmful to us, so we spit it out and stop drinking it. The body also uses the bowel and bladder systems to excrete micro-organisms in the form of urine and faeces.

HOW ARE MICRO-ORGANISMS SPREAD?

Micro-organisms can be spread through six potential routes, which are listed below:

1. Direct contact
2. Indirect contact
3. Airborne route
4. Faecal–oral route
5. Animal vector
6. Bloodborne route

Direct contact can come from person to person through kissing or sexual contact. Indirect contact can spread micro-organisms through contaminated hands coming in contact with another surface or person. Micro-organisms can be spread via the airborne route from a person sneezing or coughing near another person or through the disturbance of dust when cleaning. Microbes can also be spread via the faecal–oral route from humans to humans through poor hand hygiene – for example, not washing your hands after going to the toilet and then proceeding to prepare food. The microbes are spread to the food preparation area and then can be ingested when it is eaten. Animal vector, such as mosquitoes, can bite through the skin and insert micro-organisms into the body, which cause malaria. Micro-organisms can be spread via the blood-borne route through the sharing of dirty, used equipment or through the spread of infected blood or bodily fluids that may be splashed onto another person.

THE CHAIN OF INFECTION

There are six links in the chain of infection. These are as follows:

1. Causative agent
2. Reservoir
3. Portal of exit
4. Transmission
5. Portal of entry
6. Susceptible host

Figure 2.1 shows us each individual link with its corresponding stage in the process of infection prevention. Understanding the characteristics of each link provides the nurse with methods to support vulnerable patients and to prevent the spread of infection and also provides the nurse with the knowledge of self-protection.

How to break the chain of infection

The method of infection prevention required is to break the chain of infection at one of the six elements. The easiest place to break the chain is to break the chain at the mode of transmission, link number 4 in Fig. 2.1. This can be done by complying with infection prevention policies and guidelines, practicing good hygiene techniques as well as good environmental cleaning practices. Figure 2.2 given below highlights several methods for breaking the chain of infection at each link.

THE FOUR AREAS OF STANDARD PRINCIPLES (SP) FOR PREVENTING HCAIs

The four areas of standard principles (SP) for preventing HCAIs are hand hygiene, use of personal protective equipment (PPE), cleaning and waste disposal. We shall now review these four areas of SP in further detail.

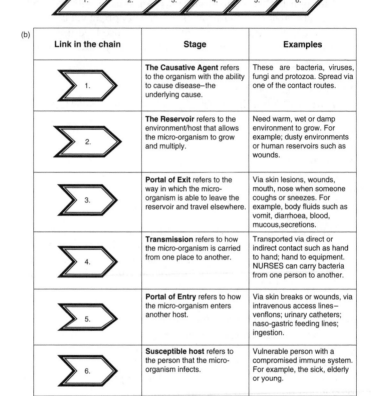

(a)

(b)

Link in the chain	Stage	Examples
1.	**The Causative Agent** refers to the organism with the ability to cause disease–the underlying cause.	These are bacteria, viruses, fungi and protozoa. Spread via one of the contact routes.
2.	**The Reservoir** refers to the environment/host that allows the micro-organism to grow and multiply.	Need warm, wet or damp environment to grow. For example; dusty environments or human reservoirs such as wounds.
3.	**Portal of Exit** refers to the way in which the micro-organism is able to leave the reservoir and travel elsewhere.	Via skin lesions, wounds, mouth, nose when someone coughs or sneezes. For example, body fluids such as vomit, diarrhoea, blood, mucous,secretions.
4.	**Transmission** refers to how the micro-organism is carried from one place to another.	Transported via direct or indirect contact such as hand to hand; hand to equipment. NURSES can carry bacteria from one person to another.
5.	**Portal of Entry** refers to how the micro-organism enters another host.	Via skin breaks or wounds, via intravenous access lines– venflons; urinary catheters; naso-gastric feeding lines; ingestion.
6.	**Susceptible host** refers to the person that the micro-organism infects.	Vulnerable person with a compromised immune system. For example, the sick, elderly or young.

Fig. 2.1 (a) Diagram of the links in the chain of infection. (b) Individual links in the chain.

Hand hygiene

To reduce HCAIs, it is essential that all healthcare workers adopt good hand hygiene practices (Nazarko, 2008). Hands are a storage area for micro-organisms to congregate, which then can be passed from person to person or person to place and cause an infection. The National Patient Safety Agency (NPSA, 2008) states that studies revealed that healthcare workers wash their hands only 40% of the

Link in the Chain	Methods to break the link
Causative Agent 1.	Health promotion programmes relating to good sanitation and cleaning practices at home and work. Healthy eating and lifestyle to maintain immune system and reduce to risk of becoming a susceptible host. When appropriate, use of antibiotics to kill micro-organisms.
Reservoir 2.	Maintaining good standards of environmental cleaning as well as personal hygiene. Use of isolation if necessary to prevent spread to others. Use of Standard Precautions.
Portal of Exit 3.	Use of Standard Precautions and isolation if necessary as well as use of respiratory etiquette, for example covering the mouth and nose when coughing or sneezing to prevent spores being spread airborne onto another person.
Mode of Transmission 4.	Good hand hygiene practices and wearing of appropriate uniform. Avoid wearing jewellery, false nails, watches, and rings. Cleaning of equipment between uses. Single use items whereever possible in the health care setting. Maintain standards of cleanliness in health care environments.
Portal of Entry 5.	Use of aseptic technique if invasive procedures necessary. Avoid use of medical devices where possible. Promote clutter free environments. Use of good hygiene practices by staff, patients and relatives.
Susceptible host 6.	Protect the vulnerable patients (elderly with declining immune system; children with underdeveloped immune system and the immunocompromised). If you are unwell, avoid contact with vulnerable patients. Use of hand hygiene and cleaning practices. Good personal hygiene reduces spread of micro-organisms to a susceptible host.

Fig. 2.2 Methods of breaking the chain of infection.

time. Healthcare workers are the biggest risk to their patients because they have the best potential of being the mode of transmission. This is because their hands can

- transfer the patients' own micro-organisms into another part of their body during care or treatment – for example, during surgery, changing a dressing or washing a patient;
- transfer micro-organisms from patient to patient as healthcare workers visit and treat different people;
- transfer micro-organisms from the patient and the environment to another patient or another piece of equipment via direct or indirect contact;

- transfer micro-organisms from the patient to the healthcare workers during contact and can increase the risk of contracting an infection themselves.

(NPSA, 2008)

The Department of Health (DH, 2007) published guidance regarding staff uniform policy. Each NHS trust or primary care trust (PCT) will have its own policy relating to uniforms. However, one universal message from the guidance is that all staff, including medical staff, must be bare below the elbow. This means that staff should not wear long-sleeved clothing and should not wear ties, wrist watches, hand jewellery or false nails within the clinical area or point of care.

The *point of care* is the crucial time for hand hygiene. According to NPSA (2008), the point of care is defined as the patient's immediate environment (zone) where contact or treatment is taking place. Point of care could be in a patient's home, community clinic or GP practice or at the patient's bedside when in hospital. The point of care also represents the time and place where there is the highest risk for the transmission of infection via healthcare staff whose hands can act as reservoirs to transfer micro-organisms. So how do healthcare workers decide when is the right time to wash and dry their hands?

The World Health Organisation (WHO, 2006) suggests that there are five moments when hand hygiene should be performed. These are as follows:

- Before patient contact
- Before an aseptic task
- After body fluid exposure risk
- After patient contact
- After contact with patient surroundings

Let us look at these five areas in further detail. Before patient contact refers to before touching a patient; hand hygiene reduces the risk of transfer of micro-organisms from staff to patient, which may be harmful. Before an aseptic task refers to protecting the patient from the transfer of any harmful micro-organisms that may be on the staff or the patient. There is the need to reduce the risk of the micro-organisms getting inside the body and causing infection. After body fluid exposure risk refers to protecting the environment, staff and patients from any potential spread of harmful micro-organisms that cause cross-infection. After patient contact is necessary because micro-organisms from the patients and their surroundings could be transferred onto staff and then spread elsewhere and cause infection in other staff and patients. After contact with patient surroundings relates to protecting yourself, your colleagues and other patients as well as the healthcare environment from exposure to harmful micro-organisms.

So how should you clean your hands?

It cannot be emphasised enough how such a simple thing as washing your hands can reduce and prevent infection. Healthcare workers are encouraged to use either soap and water or alcohol hand rubs. The technique for cleaning hands is the same irrespective of the product used.

The NHS principles for hand washing are based on the six-stage hand washing technique (Aycliffe et al., 1978), although different hospitals may have adapted this to include more stages. The Pennine Acute Hospitals Trust in Greater Manchester, for example, has a seven-stage approach. It is important that if using the soap and water technique, you wet your hands first and then apply the liquid soap. Then follow the seven stages that are listed below:

1. Wash palm to palm.
2. Wash palm over back of hand with interlocking fingers – then swap hands and repeat.
3. Wash palm to palm with interlocking fingers.
4. Rub the back of the fingers into the palm of the hands.
5. Wash the thumbs using a rotational movement clasped over opposite palm – then swap hands and repeat for the other thumb.
6. Wash the palm of each hand by rotationally rubbing the fingers into the palm – then swap hands and repeat.
7. Wash around wrists using rotational rubbing with clasped hand – then swap hands and repeat for opposite wrists.

The whole procedure will take between 15 and 30 seconds.

There are many posters and pictures of the stages of hand washing technique in hospitals and community clinics to assist people to use the correct technique. If you want to see hand washing demonstrated in video action, the NPSA website (www.npsa .nhs.uk/cleanyourhands) also has a video that can be watched. Alternatively, you can look at the pictures below and practice the technique. Using the correct hand washing technique is very important and many NHS hospitals are assessing their staff to ensure they are using the correct technique (Fig. 2.3).

You may use alcohol hand rubs as an alternative to soap and water. The use of alcohol hand rub is suggested for use in all patient care settings except in the following circumstances. These are when hands are visibly soiled, when the patient has diarrhoea and/ or vomiting, when there is direct hand contact with bodily fluids and when there is an occurrence of diarrhoeal sickness such as Norovirus or *Clostridium Difficile*.

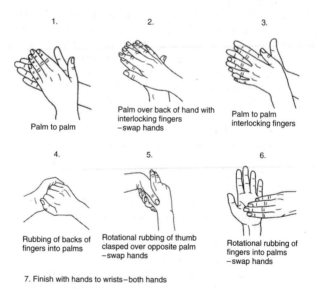

1.

Palm to palm

2.

Palm over back of hand with interlocking fingers
−swap hands

3.

Palm to palm interlocking fingers

4.

Rubbing of backs of fingers into palms

5.

Rotational rubbing of thumb clasped over opposite palm −swap hands

6.

Rotational rubbing of fingers into palms −swap hands

7. Finish with hands to wrists−both hands

Fig. 2.3 The seven stages of the hand washing technique.

Practice point 2.1

What practical steps can be taken to ensure that when there is an outbreak of diarrhoea that everyone (patient, staff and visitors) in the healthcare environment uses the soap and water hand washing techniques?

Alcohol hand rub dispensers can either be worn by the nurse or the dispensers be placed at the point of care within the acute hospital setting. It is important that a risk assessment of the environment be completed when deciding where to place the dispensers, especially if the healthcare setting includes children, mental health patients and confused and vulnerable adults.

To maintain the good condition of the hands and reduce the risk of exacerbating any skin problems such as contact dermatitis, nurses and other healthcare workers must ensure that they wash and dry their hands properly and use hand moisturisers that will be provided through their employer. Staff may contact their occupational health departments for advice regarding hand care.

Aseptic non-touch technique

Another method to reduce the risk of cross-infection and spread of micro-organisms is to apply the aseptic non-touch technique (ANTT) when carrying out procedures such as glucose sampling, venepuncture, cannulation or even changing of feeding bags. ANTT is a robust, efficient and evidence-based aseptic technique and it has been shown to significantly reduce HCAI as well as improve the clinical practice of staff performing aseptic procedures. The principle of this is not to touch the 'key parts' that will come in contact with each other. For example, when preparing for venepuncture, the syringe tip should only touch the hub of the needle and nothing else. Many organisations have posters to display the principles of ANTT as an acronym.

Always wash hands
Non-touch technique to protect key parts
Touch non-key parts with confidence
Take appropriate infection prevention (IP) precautions

Use of personal protective equipment (PPE)

Using PPE is one of the standards for infection prevention. PPE is a collective term that refers to the use of disposable gowns, aprons, masks, goggles/visors and gloves by healthcare workers at work when dealing with patients. It is also part of the health and safety rules and regulations of the United Kingdom. Employers and employees are expected to know these rules and abide by them.

The government regulations dictate that PPE falls into the Health and Safety at Work Act (1974) and the Control of Substances Hazardous to Health (COSHH) (Health and Safety Executive (HSE) 2002). The law states that healthcare workers and employers must recognize and manage any hazard risks in the workplace. The NHS and private sector have to comply with the law of the land and therefore provide healthcare workers with PPE. Equally, healthcare workers are expected to think about their own personal health and safety as well as the safety of patients and use the PPE provided. PPE should be easily accessible for all staff, whatever the healthcare environment they are working in.

Infection prevention using gloves

To reduce the risk of micro-organisms being spread from person to person, gloves are an essential PPE that protect nurses from being infected by micro-organisms found in blood, sputum, vomit, diarrhoea, leaking wounds, drains or urinary catheters. Gloves should be used at the point of care and during contact and not be worn elsewhere. After use, the gloves themselves will have become contaminated with micro-organisms and so must be removed and disposed of immediately in a clinical waste bin. Hands must be cleaned after the removal of the gloves before leaving the point of care area to prevent infection, as micro-organisms will have multiplied, spreading through contact with another patient or colleague. Wearing the same pair of gloves from patient to patient is an infection hazard. Changing gloves and washing your hands after each patient is essential in order to prevent micro-organisms from being transferred from person to person.

Gloves can either be sterile or non-sterile. Nurses and healthcare workers need to assess the 'infection risk' in each situation they are in to decide which type of glove is required.

Practice point 2.2

Consider the following examples and think about whether the use of sterile or non-sterile gloves is the most appropriate PPE. Tick the box that you decide is the correct answer.

Clinical activity	Sterile gloves	Non-sterile gloves	No gloves
Washing the patient's hands and face			
Emptying the urinary catheter			
Aspiration of percutaneous endoscopic gastrotomy (PEG) feeding line and changing feed			
Changing a leg ulcer wound dressing			
Cleaning and changing a stoma bag			
Cleaning up vomit that has come in contact with the bed clothes			
Emptying a urinal full of urine			
Emptying a commode full of urine and faeces			
Changing the dressing around a peripheral venflon site			
Changing the dressing around a tracheostomy stoma site			
Assisting the awake patients to brush their teeth			
Providing eye care to the unconscious patient			

Infection prevention using aprons

Disposable aprons will protect your uniform and reduce the risk of transferring any micro-organisms from patient to patient. Aprons will also protect you from coming into contact with bodily fluids that may be unintentionally splashed onto you. Aprons should be worn where there is close direct contact with the patients and their defined point of care environment. The defined area may include any additional equipment such as feeding pumps, infusion pumps, drip stands, lockers, tables or chairs. If you are a nurse who works in a hospital ward area, it is also important that at meal times, when serving food an apron is worn. Some areas use colour-coded aprons that indicate that food is being served. It is advisable to contact your employer or access your local guidelines and policies regarding the standards for food hygiene practices and your local training regulations.

Practice point 2.3

Consider the following examples and think about whether sterile, non-sterile or no aprons are required. Tick the box that you think is the correct answer.

Clinical activity	No apron required	Sterile apron	Non-sterile apron
Bed bathing a patient			
Changing sheets on a bed			
Giving out meals			
Cleaning a bed area from a discharged patient			
Answering the telephone			
Changing a stoma bag			
Recording physiological observations			
Cleaning a drip stand			

When the nurse assists the doctor with sterile, invasive procedures it may be necessary for staff to use a sterile, single use, fluid repellent gown. These gowns are pre-packed, disposable gowns that have been sterilised to decontaminate them from micro-organisms, for use in areas such as theatres or oncology.

If you are a nurse who works within the Primary Care Trust (PCT), you will have to perform a risk assessment regarding the times when you will use aprons within the homes of your patients. It is important that you do not make the patient feel uncomfortable about the use of aprons and are sensitive to their needs by explaining to them in advance why you have to use PPE.

Infection prevention using goggles or visors

Goggles and visors can protect your eyes from splashes of any airborne spray from body fluids or micro-organisms during a clinical activity, for example, a patient with projectile vomiting. It will ensure that you do not get any body fluids into your eyes and reduce the risk of eye infections. Goggles are provided by the employer, but it is the employee who must take the responsibility to choose when it is appropriate to wear them by ensuring that a risk assessment has been made to determine the use or need for goggles within specific clinical circumstances.

Infection prevention using face masks

Face masks protect the mouth and nose from accidental splashes and also prevent the nurse from inhaling any infected bodily fluids that may be sprayed into the environment – for example, a patient with infective tuberculosis (TB) who sneezes or coughs. It is vital that you protect yourself in order to stay healthy so that you can still work and care for your patients.

Some patients may be cared for within single rooms or side rooms within the ward area. A key point when using face masks as a PPE is to put the mask on before contact with the patient, before entering the single room and then being careful about which areas of the mask (or apron) you touch. Remove and discard the face mask with care, ensuring that the front of the face mask (or apron) is not touched because this is the highest contact risk area. Place used PPE in the yellow clinical waste bins and wash your hands thoroughly before leaving the point of care area.

Cleaning

A clean environment will drastically reduce the risk of HCAI for our patients. Therefore, it is important that high standards of cleanliness are maintained by all staff who work in a healthcare setting. However, nurses may delegate to students or support workers roles of cleaning and decontamination of equipment. An example of this would be cleaning and changing bed linen or bed areas in order to reduce the amount of dust and therefore the amount of micro-organisms in the environment. Other factors that require standards of cleanliness to reduce the amount of dirt and dust and prevent the risk of accidents are to minimise the accumulation of clutter in the surrounding areas.

Most routine cleaning can be carried out using the damp dusting method. This is when soap and water are used to clean the flat surfaces of equipment and then thoroughly dried. A damp surface only encourages the micro-organisms to grow because, as discussed earlier, they like heat and moisture to multiply.

Each NHS hospital, private or PCT, has guidelines that relate to cleaning and infection prevention. A colour coding system is used to guide staff on which cloths to use in which type of environment.

Practice point 2.4

An elderly gentleman arrives at the community clinic for his podiatry appointment. He is asked by the staff to take a seat in the waiting room while he waits to be called in to see the podiatrist. He suddenly gets up and asks for directions to the toilet but unfortunately on his way, he is unable to control his bowels and is incontinent of faeces. He is extremely upset and distressed.

Having read this chapter, indicate what *infection prevention* measures should be taken in relation to the needs of (a) the gentleman (b) other patients waiting for their podiatry appointment and (c) the staff?

When a patient who has had a serious infection leaves the clinical setting, the environment will need to be decontaminated using the guidelines for deep or terminal cleaning before any new patient can be admitted (Pratt et al., 2007). If there has been a virulent strain of infection on the ward where two or more patients have been infected, then the infection prevention team may request a deep or terminal clean. The deep clean would include the changing of curtains, washing of walls, cleaning behind radiators, the internal windows and horizontal surfaces as well as changing or cleaning the mattress on the bed. In areas where there are carpets in use, such as nursing homes, the carpets would require steam cleaning. Most clinical areas have now changed to floor and furniture that is easy to wash and does not collect dust. The deep clean guidelines would be used following an outbreak of infection in a clinical setting, for example, Norovirus or *Clostridium*. Once the deep or terminal cleaning has been completed, it is safe to readmit patients to the area.

Safe use and disposal of sharps and clinical waste

There may be occasions when nurses will be expected to use sharps during clinical activity – for example, obtaining blood glucose or performing venepuncture. It is recommended that sharps be single use and disposable. Sharps include items such as needles, stylets, suture needles, surgical blades, to name but a few. All sharps should be disposed of into a yellow sharps box at the point of use. The regulations for the yellow sharps box are defined as 'non-permeable, puncture-resistant, tamper-proof container' (Royal College of Nursing (RCN), 2007, p. 13) and should comply with British Standards. Sharps boxes should be easily accessible and positioned as near the clinical procedure area as is practically possible (Pratt et al., 2007). Sharps should be disposed of by the user and staff should not overfill the containers by filling then only to the designated line marked on the box. This equates to no more than 75% of its maximum capacity. Sharps bins should be secured and positioned at a height that enables all members of the clinical team to dispose of their sharps safely and easily but also out of reach of children.

Sharps should not be handled directly and should be disposed of after clinical use in the yellow sharp bins provided by the employer. It is not acceptable to put sharps or clinical waste in black plastic waste sacks. Yellow clinical bags should not be overfilled, as this can create a manual handling risk to waste disposal handlers such as portering staff. When disposing of clinical waste, care should be taken to protect and maintain the immediate environment from contamination as well as ensuring safety of those who come into contact with waste (Blenkharn, 2009a).

According to Blenkharn (2009a), there are regular problems with inappropriate items being disposed of in black waste sacks instead of the yellow clinical waste sacks or sharps bins. Examples include blood and body fluids not emptied from drainage bags, chest drain bottles, urinary catheters and dialysis fluid. This puts ancillary and support staff as well as commercial waste contractors at high risk of accidental injury or harm. Blenkharn (2009a) suggests that there is little thought by clinical staff about the welfare of others who may come into contact with clinical waste as it passes along the disposal chain. He calls for a change in practices with regard to protective work wear such as reinforced puncture and cut-resistant panels to trousers and gloves. Unfortunately, within the healthcare setting, most ancillary staff who handle clinical waste containers will only be provided with disposable gloves and these offer no protection from penetrating injury. Studies have found that almost 100% of waste handlers' clothing becomes contaminated with blood splashes within 4 hours of commencing work (Blenkharn, 2009b).

Despite guidance that resheathing of needles should not occur, it accounts for 51% of needle stick injuries among nurses (RCN, 2007). Sharps must not be recapped, bent, broken or dismantled after use (Pratt et al., 2007). There should be guidance provided by your employer regarding the safe use and disposal of sharps. Ball and Pike (2008) found that within NHS settings, 96% of nurses reported that there was a sharps policy that covered prevention and reporting of needle stick injury, but in non-NHS settings, only 81% had a policy.

Ball and Pike (2008) were commissioned by the Royal College of Nursing (RCN) to do a postal and an online survey of needle stick injuries with 4407 nurses responding the survey. Forty-eight percent had been stuck by a needle or sharp at some point in their career and 10% had been injured within the last year. According to the report, many of these injuries would not have an adverse effect; however, the psychological harm from worrying about whether or not the nurse has been infected with diseases such as hepatitis B, hepatitis C or HIV is immeasurable.

Gabriel (2009) outlines four areas for prevention of sharp-related injuries. These include risk assessment, procedures and policies, safe systems of work and incident reporting. Employers are obliged to carry out risk assessments for staff who are at risk of being exposed to infectious bodily fluids or materials that may be hazardous to health. Employers are also expected to put policies and procedures in place to prevent sharp-related incidents from occurring. These policies and procedures should be easily accessible for staff and are identified by the bright yellow (hazard warning colour) files they are kept in.

Pratt et al. (2007) outlined within the epic2 document that avoiding sharp-related injuries is everybody's responsibility. Staff and employers are both responsible for safety and staff should be encouraged to report sharps injuries. This information is then collected by the EPINet™ surveillance project. The use of needlefree or protective devices has been suggested to be another way of reducing injuries (Pratt et al., 2007; Gabriel, 2009). Should a needle stick or sharps injuries occur, the area should be allowed to bleed and washed under running water for at least 2 minutes and the nurses should remember not to suck the area of injury (Dougherty and Lamb, 2008). Any areas of the skin that have cuts or abrasions should be covered with a blue coloured, waterproof dressing. It should be reported to a senior member of staff for support and advice.

CONCLUSION

HCAIs cost the NHS an estimated £1 billion a year because of the impact of longer periods of illness, stay in hospital and the expense of treatments. The leading HCAIs found in the community and hospital settings are urinary tract infections and the second most common HCAIs are lower respiratory tract infections. Not all HCAIs can be prevented, but it is estimated that between 15% and 30% are preventable. Unfortunately, the most common cause for the spread of HCI is the contaminated hands of healthcare workers, medical equipment and failure of staff to comply with local policies, procedures and guidelines.

These guidelines are based on national recommendations, commissioned by the Department of Health. In the acute setting, the epic2 guidelines were published through *The Journal of Hospital*

37

Infection (Pratt et al., 2007). The guidelines for primary and community care are called 'Infection control: Prevention of health care-associated infection in primary and community care' and published by the *British Journal of Infection Control* (Pellowe et al., 2003). Infection prevention should be the concern of everybody from patient, relative, nurse, doctor and, importantly for you, the healthcare worker. Remember, CLEAN HANDS SAVE LIVES (NPSA, 2008). A really useful website to access about infection prevention is www.infectioncontrol.nhs.uk.

REFERENCES

Aycliffe GA, Babbo JR, Quoraishi AH (1978). A test for 'hygienic' hand disinfection. *Journal of Clinical Pathology* **31**(10), 913–928.

Ball J and Pike J (2008). *Needlestick Injury in 2008. Results from a Survey of RCN Members.* London, Royal College of Nursing.

Blenkharn J (2009a). Sharps management and the disposal of clinical waste. *British Journal of Nursing* **18**(14), 860–864.

Blenkharn J (2009b). Blood and body fluids exposures in clinical waste handlers. *Annuals of Occupational Hygiene* **52**(4), 281–286.

Department of Health (2007). *Uniforms and Work Wear: An Evidence Base for Developing Local Policy.* London, Department of Health.

Department of Health (2008). *The Health Act 2006: Code of Practice for the Prevention and Control of Health Care Acquired Infections.* London, Department of Health.

Dougherty L and Lamb J (2008). *Intravenous Therapy in Nursing Practice.* 2nd edn. Oxford, Blackwell Publishing Ltd.

Gabriel J (2009). Reducing needlestick and sharps injuries among healthcare workers. *Nursing Standard* **23**(22), 41–44.

Health and Safety at Work Act (1974). http://www.hse.gov.uk/legislation/hswa.htm [Accessed 15th January 2010].

Health and Safety Executive (HSE) (2002). *The Control of Substances Hazardous to Health Regulations 2002. Approved Code of Practice and Guidance L5.* 4th edn. London, Health and Safety Executive.

National Patient Safety Agency (NPSA) (2008). *Clean Hands Save Lives. Patient Safety Alert.* 2nd edn., 2nd September 2008.

Nazarko L (2008). Standard precautions: how to help prevent infection. *British Journal of Health Care Assistants* **2**(33), 119–123.

Oxford Dictionary (2008). *Concise Oxford English Dictionary.* 11th edn..

Pellowe CM, Pratt RJ, Harper P, et al. (2003). Infection control: prevention of health-care associated infection in primary and community care. *Journal of Hospital Infection* **55**, S2–S3.

Pratt RJ, Pellowe CM, Wilson JA, et al. (2007). Epic 2: National evidence-based guidelines for preventing healthcare-associated infections in NHS Hospitals in England. *Journal of Hospital Infection* **65**(Suppl. 1), S1–S64.

Royal College of Nursing (RCN) (2007). *Standards for Infusion Therapy*. London, RCN IV Therapy Forum.
World Health Organisation (WHO) (2006). *Your 5 Moments for Hand Hygiene*. Version 1. Geneva, WHO.

USEFUL WEBSITES
www.npsa.nhs.uk/cleanyourhands
www.infectioncontrol.nhs.uk
www.hpa.org.uk
www.hse.gov.uk

APPENDIX
Useful examples of adapted Infection Prevention Guidelines reprinted courtesy of Pennine Acute NHS Trust, Greater Manchester.

Emptying a urine collection bag
A clean technique with gloves and aprons worn as PPE

Equipment
1. Non-sterile gloves
2. Apron
3. 2% Chlorhexidine and 70% alcohol wipe × 2
4. Disposable urine bottle – male type, or disposable jug
5. Clinical waste bag

Procedure

Step	Action	Rationale
	Explain and discuss procedure with the patient to reassure and obtain consent	
1.	Clean hands with soap and water or alcohol hand rub using 7-stage technique	Remove transient bacteria
2.	Apply gloves and apron and consider the need for face masks or goggles	To protect self from potential urine spillage and splash

(continued)

Continued

Step	Action	Rationale
3.	With urine bag hanging on stand (ensuring that it does not touch the floor), place bag outlet into disposable urine bottle	To prevent splashing of urine and cross contamination
4.	Clean valve using alcohol wipe. Allow to dry. Then open the valve and allow urine to empty without lifting urine bag	Lifting bag can cause reflux of urine into bladder and increase potential of UTI
5.	When bag is empty, shut valve. Clean outlet with chlorhexidine and alcohol wipe and allow to dry. Place used wipe in clinical waste bag	To remove transient bacteria – Decontamination occurs when surface has dried. To prevent splashing of urine
6.	Remove disposable urine bottle to sluice. Weigh if necessary. Dispose of urine bottle and contents into macerator	Safe waste management
7.	Remove gloves and apron and dispose of all clinical waste	Safe waste management
8.	Clean hands with soap and water or alcohol hand rub using 7-stage technique	Remove transient bacteria
9.	Document output if necessary	Maintain fluid balance record

Note: Routine daily personal hygiene is all that is needed to maintain meatal hygiene. Maintain a closed system and only empty bag when necessary. Do not allow to overfill to prevent reflux occurring.
Always keep bag off the floor and below the level of the bladder, to reduce cross-infection and urine draining back into bladder causing infection.

Obtaining a catheter specimen of urine (CSU) using an aseptic non-touch technique

A clean technique with low risk of touching key parts therefore non-sterile gloves are used with disposable non-sterile aprons worn as PPE.

Equipment

1. Procedure tray or trolley
2. Non-sterile gloves and disposable apron
3. 2% Chlorhexidine and 70% alcohol wipe × 2
4. Gate clamp
5. 20 ml luer slip syringe
6. Alcohol hand rub
7. Urine specimen collection pot
8. Sharps bin
9. Waste bag
10. Eye protection

Procedure

Step Action	Rationale
Explain and discuss the procedure with the patient to reassure and obtain consent	
1. Clean hands with soap and water or alcohol hand rub using 7 stage technique	Remove transient bacteria
2. Apply non-sterile gloves and apron	PPE
3. Clean tray with Chlorhexidine and alcohol wipe from the inside to outside of tray/trolley	To provide an aseptically clean work surface
Remove PPE and decontaminate hands	
Apply new apron and gloves	

(continued)

Continued

Step	Action	Rationale
4.	Open syringe and leave in opened packet	To protect key part of syringe
	Place into tray	
	Place other equipment into tray	
5.	Take tray and equipment to patient's bedside	
6.	Check patient details with specimen request card	Ensure correct diagnostic test for patient
	Expose sampling port	
7.	Only if there is no urine in the tubing, clamp the tubing with the gate clamp below the access port on catheter bag	To ensure sufficient urine for collection
8.	Remove and dispose of gloves and apron. Wash hands using 7 stage hand washing technique or clean hands with alcohol rub using 7 stage technique	To remove transient bacteria
9.	Put on new non-sterile gloves and apron	Low risk of touching key parts and PPE
10.	Clean the sampling port with chlorhexidine and alcohol wipe	To remove transient bacteria from this key part
	Allow to dry	Decontamination occurs when surface has dried
	Place used wipe in waste bag	

Continued

Step	Action	Rationale
11.	*Needleless sampling port:* insert the syringe firmly into the centre of the sampling port (following manufacturer's instructions). Aspirate the required amount of urine and disconnect the syringe	To reduce the risk of needlestick injury
12.	Remove specimen collection pot lid	Prevent spillage of any residual urine
	Transfer urine sample from syringe into collection bottle	
	Dispose of syringe as per waste policy	
13.	Replace specimen collection pot lid securely	Prevent spillage
14.	Remove gloves and apron and dispose of all waste	Safe waste management
15.	Clean hands with soap and water or alcohol hand rub using 7 stage technique	Remove transient bacteria
16.	Complete details of specimen collection pot label. Document sample collection.	Ensure correct diagnostic test for patient. Record event
17.	Remove procedure trolley from bedside and dispose of all waste	

Topical applications – MRSA eradication treatment

A clean procedure with low risk of touching key parts therefore non-sterile gloves are used with disposable aprons worn as PPE.

Equipment

1. Suitable clean surface
2. Washing bowl with water
3. Topical applications – skin wash, nasal cream and mouthwash
4. Apron
5. Non-sterile gloves
6. Washing wipes
7. Clinical waste bag
8. Alcohol hand rub
9. Red bag

Procedure

Step	Action	Rationale
1.	Explain procedure to patient and answer any questions sensitively and ensure patient has information leaflet for reference	Reassurance because the patient may be worried and concerned about colonization and its consequences
	Refer any difficulties to senior staff	
2.	Clean hands with soap and water or alcohol hand rub using 7 stage technique	Remove transient bacteria
3.	Apply non-sterile gloves and apron	PPE
4.	Wet the patient's skin	

Continued

Step	Action	Rationale
5.	Pour about 30ml of skin wash onto dry wipe and rub into patient's skin for 1 minute. Cover as wide an area as is possible at a time but ensure the patient doesn't get cold.	Skin wash to be allowed to sit on skin for 1 min.
	If bed bathing ensure all areas are washed paying particular attention to axilla, groin and perineal areas. Hair to be washed twice a week. If patient is self-caring, wash back and any other parts patient cannot reach. Advise patient to pay particular attention to the above areas	People cannot usually reach all areas of own back
	Advise patient that wash should not be diluted into wash water or bath water	Full concentration is needed to be effective decontaminant
	Advise patient that skin wash should not be used under a running shower	Skin wash must be allowed to sit on skin for 1 minute
6.	Dry skin	Prevent excoriation
7.	Remove gloves and apron and dispose of safely	Safe waste management
8.	Clean hands with soap and water or alcohol hand rub using 7 stage technique	Remove transient bacteria
9.	Apply non-sterile gloves and apron	PPE

(continued)

Continued

Step	Action	Rationale
10.	Apply pea-sized application of nasal cream to little finger	
11.	Apply cream into front part of the inside or one nostril	Correct application of treatment
12.	Repeat into second nostril	PPE
13.	Gently press nostrils together and move fingers in a small circular motion for a moment	To disperse cream to inside of each nostril
14.	Remove gloves and apron and dispose of safely	Safe waste management
15.	Document application of topical treatment	Record keeping

Following treatment application, clean clothes, linen and towelling should be provided. *Mouthwash to be used, dentures cleaned with same. For the unconscious patient mouthwash to be used for 'mouth care'.*

Removal of peripheral IV cannula
A clean procedure using ANTT with low risk of touching key parts; therefore non-sterile gloves are used and disposable aprons worn as PPE.

Equipment
1. Clean surface – dressing trolley or tray
2. Disposable plastic apron
3. Non-sterile gloves
4. Sterile gauze

5. Sterile plaster
6. Yellow sharps bin
7. Clinical waste bag
8. Alcohol hand rub

Procedure

Step	Action	Rationale
1.	Explain the procedure to the patient and obtain his/her consent	To help reduce any anxieties the patient may have and enable him/her to cooperate
2.	Clean hands with soap and water or alcohol hand rub using 7 stage technique	Remove transient bacteria
3.	Apply non-sterile gloves and apron	PPE
4.	Clean tray with Chlorhexidine and alcohol wipe	To provide an aseptically clean work surface
5.	Open sterile gauze packet and leave gauze in packaging	
6.	Transfer equipment to patients bedside	
7.	Remove gloves/apron and dispose of	Safe waste management
8.	Clean hands with soap and water or alcohol hand rub using 7 stage technique	Remove transient bacteria
9.	Apply non-sterile gloves and apron	PPE
10.	Gently loosen existing cannula dressing	

(continued)

Continued

Step	Action	Rationale
11.	Remove gauze from packet touching one side only and place over cannula site without occluding coloured port. DO NOT apply pressure or press down on gauze	To be prepared for potential blood spillage from cannula site Prevent damage to vein
12.	Slowly remove the cannula and dressing, and check integrity before disposing in sharps bin	Check complete integrity of device before disposal. Safe waste management
13.	Once cannula is removed, apply pressure to gauze until haemostasis is achieved	Prevent haematoma
14.	Apply plaster until puncture site is closed	Protect site
15.	Remove gloves and apron and dispose	Safe waste management
16.	Clean hands with soap and water or alcohol hand rub using 7 stage technique	Remove transient bacteria
17.	Document removal in care plan, recording VIP score	Record keeping

The Respiratory System

3

INTRODUCTION

Measuring and recording the respiratory rate is a fundamental component of the patient's vital signs. It is recognised as one of the most sensitive indicators of critical illness, but it is often not completed during vital signs monitoring (McQuillan et al., 1998; National Confidential Enquiry into Patient Outcome and Death, (NCEPOD), 2005). A study by Kenward et al. (2001) advocated that nurses 'put the R back in TPR' (temperature, pulse and respiration) and revealed that only 27% of patients actually had their respiratory rate recorded on the TPR chart, although within the case notes nurses documented that the patients had increased shortness of breath (SOB). The study also found that in 52% of the cardiac arrests audited, there was a record within the case notes of increased SOB preceding cardiac arrest. The reason why the respiration rate was not recorded was explored and it was suggested that the possible factors contributing to a lack of respiratory rate observations included 'an over-reliance on technology' and the delegation of observations to the healthcare assistants (Kenward et al., 2001, p. 33). The National Institute for Health and Clinical Excellence (NICE) has called for the recording of the respiratory rate to be a mandatory measurement on the patient's observation charts (NICE, 2007).

LEARNING OUTCOMES

By the end of this chapter, you will to be able to discuss the following:

❑ The structure of the respiratory system
❑ How to perform a respiratory assessment

Vital Signs for Nurses: An Introduction to Clinical Observations, First Edition.
Joyce Smith and Rachel Roberts.
© 2011 Joyce Smith and Rachel Roberts. Published 2011 by Blackwell Publishing Ltd.

❏ The systematic approach for the assessment of the lungs based on the look, listen and feel approach

To understand why the respiratory system is important in maintaining life, it is necessary to have a basic understanding of the anatomy and physiology of the respiratory system (Fig. 3.1).

THE ORGANS INVOLVED IN RESPIRATION

The nose and its nostrils are covered by skin with fine hairs called cilia that catch and prevent any foreign materials we breathe in through our nose from entering the lungs. The nose is the first part of the respiratory passage through which the inspired air is warmed, moistened and filtered (Fig. 3.2). This is also called humidification (Waugh and Grant, 2001).

Coughing and sneezing are an important part of the body's defence mechanism. It is a protective response to an irritation of the upper airways and enables us to clear our airways of sputum (secretions/phlegm) and foreign bodies. Coughing may be a symptom of an illness and it is useful to observe what the patient coughs up by looking at the colour, texture and amount of sputum (Kennedy, 2007).

Normal sputum should look clear and transparent; however, sometimes when there is an infection, it can change colour.

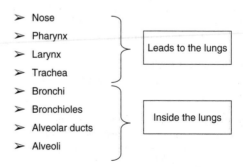

The respiratory system consists of the:

➤ Nose
➤ Pharynx
➤ Larynx   } Leads to the lungs
➤ Trachea
➤ Bronchi
➤ Bronchioles
➤ Alveolar ducts } Inside the lungs
➤ Alveoli

Fig. 3.1 The process of respiration.

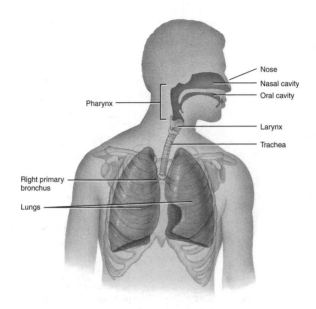

Nose
Nasal cavity
Oral cavity
Pharynx
Larynx
Trachea
Right primary bronchus
Lungs

Fig. 3.2 Anterior view of organs of respiration. Tortora and Derrickson, 2006; reprinted with permission of John Wiley and Sons Inc.

Infected sputum may look dark and green or yellow. If the patient is a smoker, the sputum may have black speckles of nicotine particles mixed in. Sometimes the sputum will look red or pink and this may indicate that there is blood present. If the sputum is frothy, it can be a sign that the lungs are waterlogged (Law, 2000; Middleton and Middleton, 2002).

The pharynx lies behind the nose and helps warm and humidify the air, as it passes through to the rest of the respiratory system. The larynx plays an important role in speech and humidification of air as it passes through. The trachea is a hollow tube that extends from the neck down into the chest and then divides into two branches called the right and left bronchi that enter both lungs (Fig. 3.3). The bronchi enter each lung where they continue to spread their branches further, becoming smaller and smaller until they become tiny bronchioles. The bronchioles look like clusters of grapes and

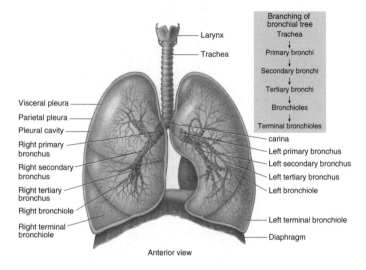

Larynx

Trachea

Visceral pleura

Parietal pleura

Pleural cavity

Right primary bronchus

Right secondary bronchus

Right tertiary bronchus

Right bronchiole

Right terminal bronchiole

Branching of bronchial tree
Trachea
↓
Primary bronchi
↓
Secondary bronchi
↓
Tertiary bronchi
↓
Bronchioles
↓
Terminal bronchioles

carina

Left primary bronchus

Left secondary bronchus

Left tertiary bronchus

Left bronchiole

Left terminal bronchiole

Diaphragm

Anterior view

Fig. 3.3 Branching of airways from the trachea: the bronchial tree. Tortora and Derrickson, 2006; reprinted with permission of John Wiley and Sons Inc.

have tiny air sacs within each grape that are called *alveoli*. This is where gaseous exchange takes place. There are two lungs that lie within the chest (thorax) on either side of the heart. The left lung is divided into two lobes (to make room for the heart space) and the right into three lobes.

For the process of breathing to happen, the ribs and sternum, which protect the lungs, work together with the diaphragm (muscles located under both lungs) and the intercostal muscles to perform the process known as *respiration* (Law and Watson, 2005).

WHAT IS THE ROLE OF THE LUNGS?

The main organ involved in respiration is the lungs. The role of the lungs is to allow exchange of gases into and out of the body. When we breathe in air we also inhale oxygen (O_2, a fuel to the body) that is used by the cells to create energy (Watson, 2000; Waugh and Grant, 2001).

The process of breathing in is known as ***inspiration;*** oxygen is transported through the alveoli and dissolves into the blood stream. When oxygen dissolves into the blood stream it attaches itself to red blood cells called *haemoglobin* (Hb), which then travel around the body delivering the oxygen to the cells. The process of creating energy within the cells is called **metabolism**. Metabolism also produces waste products – for example, carbon dioxide (CO_2) that is reabsorbed back into the lungs from the blood and disposed of through breathing out, known as **expiration** (Tortora and Derrickson, 2006; Marieb, 2009).

It is important that there is a balance between the amounts of oxygen and carbon dioxide in the body. If there is insufficient oxygen available to the cells for metabolism, the cells and tissues begin to decay. A low level of oxygen creates a condition called *hypoxia*, equally, if the body is unable to expel the carbon dioxide, the levels will increase. A high level of carbon dioxide is known as *hypercarbia*. The respiratory rate regulates the balance between the amount of oxygen and carbon dioxide to maintain homeostasis (Hickey, 2007). Factors that affect the respiration rate include respiratory diseases such as pneumonia, asthma and chronic obstructive pulmonary disease (COPD). Many conditions such as head injury, heart problems, muscular–skeletal and intestinal problems, to name but a few, may also affect the respiratory rate. Environmental and lifestyle factors such as being nervous or stressed, lack of exercise, and a poorly balanced diet with weight loss or gain may also affect the respiratory rate.

PERFORMING A RESPIRATORY ASSESSMENT

The respiratory rate is the most sensitive and important indicator when performing and recording vital signs (McQuillan et al., 1998; NICE, 2007). Ideally, prior to counting the patient's respiratory rate, the patient must rest for approximately 5 minutes (Bennett, 2003). You need to count the number of breaths per minute by looking at the chest as it rises and falls. The total number of breaths counted over 1 minute is defined as the respiration rate. In adults, the normal range is 12–20 breaths per minute and is dependant on various health factors. When counting the patient's respiratory rate it is important to observe the depth, rhythm and symmetry of the chest as it rises and falls. It is also important that the patient is not aware that you are recording their respiratory rate as they may alter their pattern of breathing.

The amount of air we breathe in and out in one breath is called the *tidal volume* (TV). To calculate an accurate TV, it requires knowledge of the patient's body weight, for example, a 50-kg patient will require a TV based on 6–10 ml/kg (The Acute Respiratory Distress Syndrome network, 2000).

$$50 \text{ kg} \times 10 \text{ ml/kg} = 500 \text{ ml}$$

Peak flow measures how much air the patient can exhale in litres per minute (Baillie et al., 2001). The chronically diseased lung over time loses it elasticity to stretch; therefore, it becomes harder for the patient to breathe in and out, and over time the lungs become stiff. One method of measuring the patients' TV is by measuring their *peak expiratory flow rate* (PEFR) using a non-invasive peak flow meter. Booker (2005) defines PEFR as a measurement of the highest rate at which air can be expelled from the lungs through an open mouth. PEFR is also included as part of the competencies in the Department of Health framework for recognising and responding to acutely ill patients (DH, 2009).

There are several ways of measuring peak flow using either a manual or an electronic meter; three consecutive PEFR readings are taken and the highest reading is then recorded. Driscoll et al. (2008) recommends that patients with asthma should have their peak flow measured in the morning and in the evening before they have their inhaled medication.

Types of breathing patterns

When observing a normal breathing pattern, it should look effortless and noiseless and the lungs should rise and fall equally on both sides (Critical Care Skills Institute (CCSI), 2009). If a person is anxious, emotionally upset or undertaking exercise, the breathing pattern may increase and is commonly known as shortness of breath. In healthy people, SOB will resolve and the breathing pattern will return to normal with rest. However, it can also be a sign that the body is not getting enough oxygen and so sometimes patients will try to compensate by increasing their RR in order to obtain more oxygen. An increase in respiratory effort is called *dyspnoea* and an increase in RR is called *tachypnoea*. There are several signs of deteriorating respiration, which include shallow, fast or slow breathing, irregular pattern, and use of accessory muscles that may potentially lead to exhaustion if no intervention is instigated. The accessory muscles used will often be the contracted muscles of the neck and shoulders and indicate that there is extra effort required to maintain breathing (Bennett, 2003).

Noisy breathing is a sign that there is a partial or total airway obstruction and is an abnormal sign. Here are a few examples that you may come across in practice. Snoring occurs when there is a partial obstruction that may be caused by the tongue. Wheezing is a high-pitched sound you may hear, which occurs when there is obstruction to your lower airways. *Stridor* is a harsh rasping sound or croaking noise that you may hear when the patient is breathing in. *Cheyne–stoke* breathing is often witnessed at the end stage of dying when the breathing pattern alternates between shallow and deep sighing breaths (Simpson, 2006).

Practice point 3.1

On a routine home visit to an elderly gentleman, he complains of feeling unwell. He informs you that he has not slept well overnight because of his breathing. He tells you he feels weak and lethargic and is coughing up green sputum.

Q1. What observations would you perform?
Q2. What action will you take following the completion of the observations?

Pulse oximetry (oxygen saturations)

Pulse oximetry is a non-invasive way of recording the pulse rate and peripheral oxygen saturation (Walters, 2007). A simple way to find out whether breathing supplies enough oxygen to the body is to monitor and record the patient's oxygen saturations. Pulse oximetry is considered a necessary component of routine vital signs monitoring (NICE, 2007). The pulse oximeter measures the percentage of Hb saturated with oxygen (O_2). This is more commonly known and recorded as SpO_2. Therefore, SpO_2 is the amount of oxygen molecules carried by Hb in the blood. Hb can bind with up to four oxygen molecules and this is recognised as 100% saturated. Low levels of oxygen attached to the Hb will lead to hypoxia, which is defined as a below-normal oxygen level (Sadik et al., 2007; Brooker, 2008).

The normal range of oxygen saturation levels may vary. According to the British Thoracic Society (2008), a normal SpO_2 target is between 94 and 98% for patients with no underlying respiratory disorders. For patients with chronic chest problems such as COPD, the aim should be to achieve an SpO_2 between 88 and 92% (Driscoll et al., 2008). The pulse oximeter may become inaccurate with saturations below 90% and requires further investigation. A range below 92% may indicate inadequate amounts of oxygen and needs to be reported to a senior member of the team (Fig. 3.4).

How it works

The pulse oximeter consists of a probe that can be attached to a finger, ear lobe or toe. From the probe, there is an infrared light sensor that is able to detect how much O_2 is being carried by Hb.

Prior to attaching the probe to the patient's finger, check that the finger digits are warm and have a good circulation. Make sure that the probe is secure but not so tight that it occludes the blood supply. If the probe is left on for too long, it may cause tissue

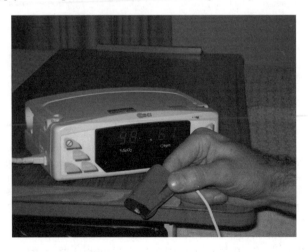

Fig. 3.4 Pulse oximetry. From Dougherty and Lister (2008).

damage; therefore, the probe needs to be rotated onto a different site. When observing for an accurate SpO_2 reading, you need to look for a good waveform trace displayed on the monitor that correlates with the pulse rate. Ensure that the alarm parameters are set according to the needs of the patient. Factors that may prevent an accurate reading include nail varnish, false nails, bright lights, poor position of probe, skin colour and poor circulation (Kennedy, 2007). A limitation of pulse oximeters is that they measure only the oxygen levels and not carbon dioxide or acid–base balance. To obtain a holistic assessment of the patient's respiratory status, further clinical observations and blood gases are required (Brooker, 2008).

Practice point 3.2

A young 20-year-old woman, who is a known asthmatic, admits herself to accident and emergency (A&E) because she is having difficulty with her breathing. She has taken her inhalers to no relieving effect.

Q1. What is the most important observation to be performed?
Q2. What other secondary observations should be performed?
Q3. What action will you take following the completion of the observations?

To be able to assess a person's RR correctly and accurately, a systematic approach needs to be used. This systematic approach is known as *Look, Listen and Feel*.

Look at the patient

Looking at your patient will help provide *visual information* that is important for your respiratory assessment to establish what is normal or abnormal. As soon as you approach the patient, you can begin the respiratory assessment by looking for visible signs of breathlessness, distress and anxiety associated with breathing; you are already gathering vital assessment clues. Observe the patient's ability to talk and engage in conversation. The ability to converse indicates that the airway is clear and patent. If the patient is using supplemental oxygen via a face mask or portable oxygen (Simpson, 2006), this may be a result of a chronic respiratory problem or it may be a new need for supplemental oxygen.

Look at the patient's skin colour

You may have heard of the terms peripheral or central *cyanosis* and this relates to sufficient oxygen being supplied to the tissue and major organs. Cyanosis has been defined as dusky or bluish tinge to the skin (Cox and McGrath, 1999). Peripheral cyanosis occurs when there is reduced oxygen being supplied to the peripheral tissue because the body is trying to conserve oxygen supply to the major organs. Finger tips and hands may look pale and feel cool to touch. Central cyanosis is a late and potential dangerous sign of poor supply of oxygenated blood to major organs and is assessed by looking at the colour of the tongue and lips.

If there is enough oxygen circulating in the body, then the patient will have a good skin colour. Sometimes the skin looks red and flushed due to changes in the blood vessels caused by problems such as high blood pressure or a severe infection.

Look at the patient's position

The position of the patient can also influence the RR, rhythm and depth. A patient who is sat upright will be able to expand the lungs better than when they are lying flat. It is important to assess the patient's current position to see whether it is affecting the breathing pattern. As part of the respiratory assessment, it is essential to note the position of the patient by observing whether they are sat up, lying down, on their side, leaning forward or appear uncomfortable (Dean, 2002).

Listening to the patient

Listening to your patient will help provide *audible information* that is important for your respiratory assessment. In normal respiration, there is no audible noisy breathing. However, in abnormal noisy breathing, you may hear sounds such as gurgling, wheezing or rattling noises that may put the airway at risk and need further interventions such as suctioning, nebulisers or physiotherapy.

Feel

Therapeutic touch of the patient's skin on the hand or arm will help provide *sensory information* to establish what is normal or abnormal. Normal skin will feel warm and soft if the circulation is good. Abnormal signs may be cold, clammy or sweaty because of hypotension and shock. By placing your hands on the patient's chest (with consent), you will be able to feel the chest rise and fall. If only one side of the chest is rising, the patient may have a consolidation of the lungs or a *pneumothorax*. This may require urgent intervention by a senior member of the team or referral for physiotherapy.

CONCLUSION

Within this chapter, we have discussed the anatomy and physiology of the respiratory system. A basic knowledge of how the lungs work aids in performing a respiratory assessment competently. Throughout this chapter, we have emphasised that the respiratory rate is the most sensitive indicator for signs of physiological deterioration in your patient. Observing and recording the respiratory rate, rhythm and depth using the look, listen and feel approach will provide a comprehensive assessment. Pulse oximeters are a useful aid in assessment, but there are limitations to their use when the patient's oxygen saturation is below 90%. Blood gases may be taken to gain clinical information but this is a specialised skill. It is essential to record the patient's respiratory rate as it is identified as a sensitive indicator and an early sign of any physiological deterioration.

REFERENCES

The Acute Respiratory Distress Syndrome Network (2000). Ventilation with lower tidal volumes as compared with traditional tidal volumes for acute lung injury and the acute respiratory distress syndrome. *The New England Journal of Medicine* **342**(18), 1301–1308.

Baillie L, Corbin V, and Higham, C (2001). Respiratory care: assessment and interventions. In: *Developing Practical Nursing Skills*, Baillie L (ed). London, Arnold, 285–332.

Bennett C (2003). Nursing the breathless patient. *Nursing Standard* **17**(17), 45–51.

Booker R (2005). Best practice in the use of spirometry. *Nursing Standard* **19**(48), 49–54.

Brooker R (2008). Pulse oximetry. *Nursing Standard* **22**(30), 39–41.

Cox CL and McGrath A (1999). Respiratory assessment in critical care units. *Intensive and Critical Care Nursing* **15**, 226–234.

Critical Care Skills Institute (CCSI) (2009). *Acute Illness Management. AIM Course Manual*. Greater Manchester Critical Care Skills Institute.

Dean E (2002). Effects of positioning and mobilization. In: *Physiotherapy for Respiratory and Cardiac Problems Adults and Paediatrics*, Pryor JA and Prasad SA (eds). London, Churchill Livingstone.

Department of Health (2009). *Competencies for Recognising and Responding to Acutely Ill Patients in Hospital*, http://www.dh.gov.uk/publications [Accessed November 2009].

Dougherty L and Lister S (2008). *The Royal Marsden Hospital Manual of Clinical Procedures*, 7th edn. Oxford, Wiley-Blackwell.

Driscoll BR, Howard LS, and Davison AG on behalf of the British Thoracic Society (2008). BTS guideline for emergency oxygen use in adult patients. *Thorax* **63** (Suppl. 6), 1–12. www.brit-thoracic.org.uk

Hickey S (2007). An audit of oxygen therapy on a respiratory ward. *British Journal of Nursing* **16**(18), 1132–1136.

Kennedy S (2007). Detecting changes in the respiratory status of ward patients. *Nursing Standard* **21**(49), 42–46.

Kenward G, Castle N, and Hodgetts T (2001). Time to put the R back in TPR. *Nursing Times* **97**(40), 32–33.

Law C (2000). A guide to assessing sputum. *Nursing Times* **96**(24), 7–10.

Law C, Watson R (2005). Respiration. In: *Physiology for Nursing Practice*, Montague SE, Watson R, Herbert RA (Eds) 3rd edn. Edinburgh, Elsevier.

Marieb EN (2009). *Essentials of Human Anatomy and Physiology*. 9th edn. San Francisco, Pearson Benjamin Cummings.

McQuillan P, Pilkington A, Allan A, et al. (1998). Confidential inquiry into quality of care before admission to intensive care. *British Medical Journal* **316**, 1853–1858.

Middleton S and Middleton PG (2002). Assessment and investigation of patients' problems. In: *Physiotherapy for Respiratory and Cardiac Problems Adults and Paediatrics*, Pryor JA and Prasad SA (eds). London, Churchill Livingstone.

National Confidential Enquiry into Patient Outcome and Death (NCEPOD) (2005). An Acute Problem?, www.ncepod.org.uk [Accessed January 2008].

National Institute for Health and Clinical Excellence (NICE) (2007). *Acutely Ill Patients in Hospital: Recognition of and Response to Acute Illness in Adults in Hospital*. London, NICE.

Sadik R, Walker C, and Elliott D (2007). Respiration and circulation. In: *Foundations of Nursing Practice Leading the Way*, Hogston R and Marjoram BA (eds). London, Palgrave Macmillan.

Simpson H (2006). Respiratory assessment. *British Journal of Nursing* **15**(9), 484–487.

Tortora G and Derrickson B (2006). *Principles of Anatomy and Physiology*. 11th edn. United States of America, John Wiley and Sons Inc.

Walters T (2007). Pulse oximetry knowledge and its effects on clinical practice. *British Journal of Nursing* **16**(21), 1332–1340.

Watson R (2000). *Anatomy and Physiology for Nurses*. 11th edn. London, Bailliere Tindall, Royal College of Nursing.

Waugh A and Grant A (2001). *Ross and Wilson Anatomy and Physiology in Health and Illness*. 9th edn. London, Churchill Livingstone.

The Cardiovascular System

4

INTRODUCTION

The blood pressure (BP), pulse (P), capillary refill time (CRT) and electrocardiogram (ECG) are clinical assessments that provide the nurse with the knowledge to determine the clinical status of a patient's cardiovascular system (CVS). The importance of BP and pulse has been reiterated within the guidelines published by the National Institute for Health and Clinical Excellence (NICE, 2007) and the National Patient Safety Agency (NPSA, 2007). The guidelines from NICE (2007) endorsed by the Department of Health (DH, 2009) state that any nurse who undertakes physiological observations must be assessed and deemed competent. Therefore, to develop the performing skills required, it is essential that you have an underpinning knowledge of the anatomy and physiology of the heart and circulation.

LEARNING OUTCOMES

By the end of this chapter, you will to be able to discuss the following:

❑ The cardiovascular system
❑ How to perform a manual pulse
❑ Types of pulse patterns – what is normal/abnormal
❑ How to perform manual blood pressure
❑ How to perform capillary refill time

Vital Signs for Nurses: An Introduction to Clinical Observations, First Edition.
Joyce Smith and Rachel Roberts.
© 2011 Joyce Smith and Rachel Roberts. Published 2011 by Blackwell Publishing Ltd.

THE CARDIOVASCULAR SYSTEM (CVS)

The CVS consists of the heart, conduction and finally the circulation. The heart is a hollow, muscular, cone-shaped organ that lies between the lungs. The three layers of the heart are the pericardium, myocardium and endocardium. The three main types of blood vessels involved in the circulation are the arteries, veins and capillaries.

The layers of the heart

The heart is encased in an outer fibrous sac known as the *pericardium* that provides a tough protective membrane against other organs in the mediastinum. Between the pericardium and the heart is a potential space containing the pericardial fluid, which prevents friction as the heart beats. The myocardium is the muscle tissue of the heart and is stimulated to contract by special electrical cells within the heart to pump the blood. The inner lining of the myocardium is called the *endocardium*, which allows the *blood to flow easily over its smooth lining*. This smooth surface prevents blood from sticking and forming clots. The outer lining of the myocardium is called the *epicardium* (Waugh and Grant, 2001; Montague et al., 2005; Walsh and Crumbie, 2007).

How blood moves through the heart

The vena cava transports blood to the heart where it enters the right atrium. Blood is transported from the right atrium via the ***tricuspid*** valve into the right ventricle where the blood fills the ventricular chamber. The right ventricle then contracts, forcing blood out of the heart and into the pulmonary artery to be re-oxygenated in the lungs. The oxygenated blood returns to the left atrium. The blood is transported from the left atrium via the ***bicuspid*** valve and flows into the left ventricular chamber. The left ventricle is more muscular than the right ventricle, as it has to pump oxygenated blood around the whole body. Once the left ventricular chamber is full of blood, the left ventricle contracts and the blood is forced into the aorta. From the aorta, the blood flows to the rest of the body (Waugh and Grant, 2001; Walsh and Crumbie, 2007; Tortora and Nielsen, 2009).

Conduction of the heart

The normal trigger for the heart to contract arises from the heart being a natural pacemaker, consisting of the sinoatrial (SA) node and the atrioventricular (AV) node, which is in the top chamber (see Fig. 4.1).

The SA node sends out a regular electrical impulse, causing the atria to contract and to pump blood to the bottom chamber known as the *ventricle*. The electrical impulse then passes through to the ventricles via a 'junction box' called the *AV node*. The electrical impulse spreads into the ventricles via the purkinje fibres, causing the muscle to contract and pump out the blood. The blood from the right ventricle goes to the lungs and the blood from the left ventricle goes to the body. The electrical conduction of the heart is measured using an ECG and it can also be measured through 3, 5 or 12 lead continuous monitoring (Walsh and Crumbie, 2007; Davey, 2008).

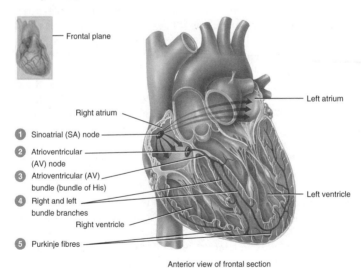

Frontal plane

Right atrium

Left atrium

1 Sinoatrial (SA) node

2 Atrioventricular (AV) node

3 Atrioventricular (AV) bundle (bundle of His)

4 Right and left bundle branches

Right ventricle

Left ventricle

5 Purkinje fibres

Anterior view of frontal section

Fig. 4.1 The conduction system of the heart. Tortora and Nielsen, 2009; reprinted with permission of John Wiley and Sons Inc.

Types of blood vessels

Once blood leaves the heart, it is transported around the body via three main blood vessels. The largest artery in the body is connected directly to the heart and is the *aorta*. Arteries transport the oxygenated blood away from the left side of the heart. Like the branches of a tree, they become thinner as they spread out from the main arteries, and as they become smaller they are called *arterioles* (Waugh and Grant, 2001; Totora and Nielsen, 2009). Imagine the blood supply around the body as a motorway system. This network has major and minor roads, just as the arteries are the major roads and the veins are the smaller side roads.

The veins transport de-oxygenated blood from all over the body back to the heart and lungs for re-oxygenation (see Fig. 4.2).

Veins are often visible just below the surface of the skin. They carry blood that is full of waste products and are de-oxygenated, which give the veins their bluish colour. The two main veins are the *inferior* and *superior vena cava*. The superior vena cava carries blood to the heart from the upper body, and the inferior vena cava carries blood to the heart from the lower body. *Capillaries* are tiny blood vessels that join on to the arterioles; they are one-cell thick and are exchanging points where the nutrients cross into the tissue cells (muscles) from the arterioles. The waste product from the tissue crosses back into the blood stream via the capillaries and then into the *venules* (Waugh and Grant, 2001; Tortora and Nielsen, 2009).

The heart has its own dedicated blood supply that is provided by the coronary arteries. While the heart is contracting, the myocardium does not receive any nutrients from the blood supply because the valves that lead to the coronary supply are closed during systole. In the resting phase (diastole), the valves open and flood the coronary arteries with blood to supply the myocardium with nutrients. The heart rate is a factor that influences the blood supply to the myocardium. The faster the heart rate, the shorter the resting time between contractions (diastole), and this can lead to signs of ischaemia, which include chest pain (angina) (Tortora and Derrickson, 2006; Marieb, 2009).

The heart pumps an average of 4–6 litres of blood around the body to the tissues every minute. This is known as cardiac output (CO). CO is influenced by the amount of blood (stroke volume, SV)

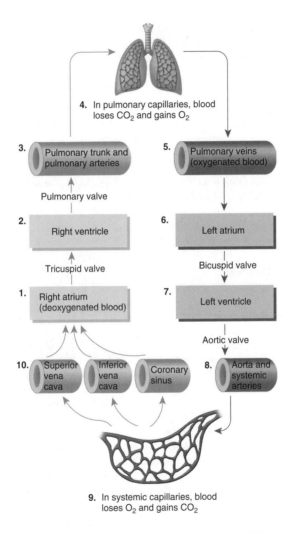

Fig. 4.2 Systemic and pulmonary circulation. Tortora and Nielsen, 2009; reprinted with permission of John Wiley and Sons Inc.

in the circulation and the heart rate (HR). It is often documented as $CO = SV \times HR$. Overall, the BP is influenced by the cardiac output and the systemic vascular resistance (SVR).

$$BP = CO \times SVR$$

CVS MONITORING

If you have an understanding of the CVS and you are competent in assessing and monitoring cardiac rhythms, you will be capable of identifying any change in the status of the heart rhythm and function (Sharman, 2007). The healthcare professional obtains measurements on the CVS using the physiological observations of pulse, BP, CRT and ECG. In order to complete a full and comprehensive assessment of the CVS, a range of cardiac investigations, for example, Urea and Electrolytes or Troponin levels, may be undertaken by healthcare professionals.

Taking the pulse

When you take the pulse, you are feeling the wave of pressure that occurs as each heartbeat causes a surge of blood circulating through the arteries. The healthcare professional will be able to palpate a pulse where the artery is close to the surface of the body (Woods et al., 2000; Waugh and Grant, 2001; Dougherty and Lister, 2008). The most frequently used site for taking a pulse is at the radial artery, although other common sites are found at the carotid, brachial and femoral arterial sites. The pulse can be affected by exercise, medication or problems with any abnormal electrical conduction of the heart. Figure 4.3 shows the main sites at which the nurse can palpate a pulse.

Checking a manual pulse is an important assessment tool that can provide information about the heart rate, the pulse pattern and how effectively the heart is pumping. Patients who are being initially assessed in the healthcare setting should have their pulse checked to provide a baseline for comparison against any new changes in the pulse pattern (Montague et al., 2005; Dougherty and Lister, 2008).

The pulse commonly taken by nurses is the radial pulse; however, when taking the patient's manual BP, you will need to use both the radial and the brachial pulses (Fig. 4.4).

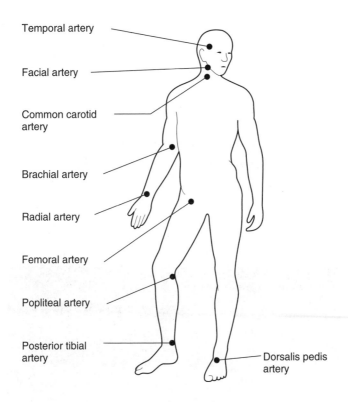

Temporal artery

Facial artery

Common carotid
artery

Brachial artery

Radial artery

Femoral artery

Popliteal artery

Posterior tibial
artery

Dorsalis pedis
artery

Fig. 4.3 Pulse points in the body. From Dougherty and Lister (2008).

A quick way to find your radial pulse is to follow the contour of the thumb towards the wrist, placing your second and third fingers on the inside of the patient's wrist. Compress your fingers until you feel the pulsation from the flow of blood through the radial artery (Fig. 4.5).

As soon as you can feel the pulse, if it is regular, best practice is to count the pulse beats for 60 seconds (Dougherty and Lister, 2008) (you will need a watch with a second hand). In practice, you may observe nurses counting the pulse for 15 seconds and then calculating the pulse by multiplying the number of beats by

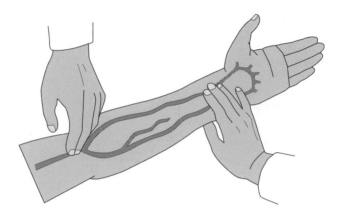

Fig. 4.4 Radial and brachial pulse.

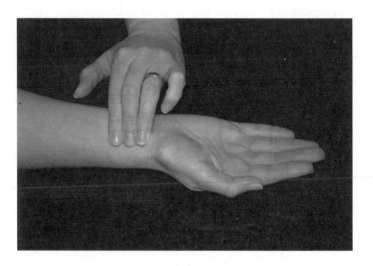

Fig. 4.5 Performing a manual pulse radial.

four. For example, 10 beats in 15 seconds (10 × 4) = 40 beats per minute (Woods et al., 2000). However, Sadik et al. (2007) state that the minimum period for counting the pulse should be 30 seconds. A normal adult resting pulse ranges from 60 to 100 beats per minute (Woods et al., 2000; Resuscitation Council UK, 2006), but this can vary because of the health and lifestyle factors of individual patients.

Practice point 4.1

What lifestyle factors affect the blood pressure?

Pulse rates may vary in different age groups, although in a healthy person the heart rate will be relatively constant (Dougherty and Lister, 2008). A regular pulse is described as a constant, consistent, rhythmic beat; but an irregular pulse is the opposite. As you read the dashes below, you can see the pattern of a regular pulse with beats represented by dashes. Notice the the beats are steady and uniform with even spacing between them as opposed to the irregular beats represented by the irregular dashes.

Regular, constant beats

‐‐‐

Irregular beats

‐‐ ‐ ‐‐ ‐ ‐ ‐‐‐ ‐ ‐ ‐ ‐‐‐ ‐ ‐ ‐

Different terminology is used in health care to describe the rate of the pulse. Common terms include the following:

- Tachycardia (pulse over 100 beats per minute)
- Bradycardia (pulse below 60 beats per minute)

However, there are cardiac patients who may have abnormal heart beats or heart rhythms. If you are unsure about the pulse rate, ensure that you discuss the findings with a member of the

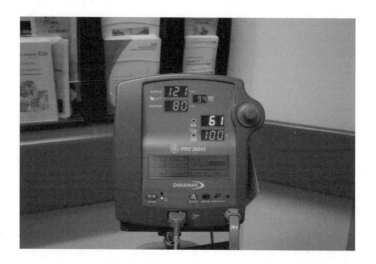

Fig. 4.6 Electronic blood pressure – a DINAMAP® machine (photograph).

healthcare team. Having obtained the pulse rate, obtaining a BP is also an important part of the assessment of the patient's cardio-vascular status and is a routine procedure that is included when monitoring the patient's vital signs.

In many healthcare settings, the use of electronic BP devices is popular – for example, a DINAMAP® machine (Fig. 4.6). These devices also display a variety of physiological data such as pulse oximetry, mean arterial pressure (MAP) and a pulse rate. However, there are limitations to obtaining information about the pulse volume and regularity from these machines. It is therefore best practice to perform a manual pulse because this will provide information about the volume and regularity of the pulse, in the assessment of an acutely unwell patient (Critical Care Skills Institute (CCSI), 2009).

The blood pressure

When your heart contracts, it pushes blood into the aorta causing an increase in pressure (systolic) and the systolic pressure is the first measurement you will record. When your heart relaxes and refills with blood, the pressure decreases (diastolic) and the last measurement is recorded. Both systolic and diastolic pressures are measured in terms of millimetres of mercury (mmHg) and both readings are known as the blood pressure (BP) and can be documented as follows:

$\dfrac{110}{70}$ *Systolic* is the top number (*Systolic* is always higher)
Diastolic is the bottom number

Another component of BP is the MAP measurement, which is an important part of the patient's physiological assessment. The MAP maybe documented on the vital signs chart. The MAP is the amount of pressure required by the body to ensure that all organs are perfused by an adequate blood supply and therefore able to function efficiently. The normal range is 70–105 (CCSI, 2009). You may have already noticed that when using an electronic BP device (Dinamap®), the MAP is displayed on the screen. It is however possible to calculate the MAP when performing a manual BP. An example is highlighted: if the BP is 180/60, you add the systolic 180 and double the diastolic 60 + 60 = 120 (180 + 120 = 300), and the total is 300; divide it by 3 (300 ÷ 3 = 100); therefore, the MAP is 100. Alternatively, for 180/60, take 60 away from 180 (180 – 60 = 120), divide 120 by 3 (120 ÷ 3 = 40) and add the 40 to the diastolic (40 + 60 = 100); the MAP is 100 (Dougherty and Lister, 2008; Marieb, 2009).

How to perform a manual non-invasive blood pressure (BP)

The three BP devices commonly used within healthcare settings are the mercury sphygmomanometer, the aneroid sphygmomanometer and the automated device (Dougherty and Lister, 2008; O'Brien, 2001). However, taking a manual BP using a stethoscope requires good hearing and interpretation. The five Korotkoff's phases are the sounds heard through the stethoscope. Table 4.1 describes what you should hear in each phase from the systolic to the diastolic. Alternatively, you may wish to access the British Hypertension Society (BHS) webpage where you will be able to watch a video on how to correctly perform a manual BP.

Phase 1 is the first sound you will hear and this is recorded as the systolic pressure, and phase 5 is the final sound you will

Table 4.1 Korotkoff's phases of the blood pressure (British Hypertensive Society, 2009).

Phase 1	The first appearance of faint, repetitive, clear tapping sounds that gradually increase in intensity for at least two consecutive beats is the systolic blood pressure
Phase 2	A brief period may follow, during which the sounds soften and acquire a swishing quality
Phase 3	The return of sharper sounds, which become crisper to regain or even exceed the intensity of phase 1 sounds. The clinical significance, if any, of phases 2 and 3 has not been established
Phase 4	The distinct, abrupt muffling sounds that become soft and blowing in quality
Phase 5	The point at which all sounds finally disappear completely is the diastolic pressure

hear and this is recorded as the diastolic pressure. However, the skill of listening for the Korotkoff's sounds is being lost because of the widespread use of electronic BP devices (Thornett, 2007). The automatic BP machines are reported to be as accurate as invasive arterial BP monitoring to a level as low as 80 mmHg systolic BP (Hassan et al., 1993). Although mercury sphygmomanometers are considered the most accurate non-invasive device, their use has been in decline because of the health and safety issues concerning mercury (Medicines and Health products Regulatory Agency (MHRA), 2001). This has led to an increased use of aneroid sphygmomanometers. By the end of 2011, the use of mercury sphygmomanometers will be phased out.

It is recommended that healthcare professionals use a 'healthy level of suspicion and check all equipment' (Bellamy et al., 2008, p. 515) for probable leaks and incorrect cuff use. Manual BP measurements should use the non-invasive cuffs, with integrated, non-removable bladders, following the reporting of two clinical case scenarios where a non-invasive cuff had the wrong size of removable bladder inserted into the wrong cuff (Bellamy et al., 2008).

The equipment required to take a manual BP are listed below:

1. Sphygmomanometer
2. Stethoscope

3. Physiological observation chart
4. Black pen

Check that the sphygmomanometer and stethoscope are in good working order prior to use (Fig. 4.7(a) and (b)). This includes the correct cuff size for the patient. The British Hypertensive Society (2009) has outlined their standards for correct sizing of cuffs (see Table 4.2).

You also need to ensure that the sphygmomanometer has been serviced regularly. There should be a sticker on the equipment with the date of the last service, and the BHS (2009) recommends that it should be done at minimum 6 monthly intervals for mercury sphygmomanometers and more frequently for aneroid sphygmomanometers. On visual check of the equipment, look for any signs of cracks or faults on the sphygmomanometer and also ensure that the reading dial is working and is set at zero.

Before commencing the procedure wash your hands, in line with infection prevention, and obtain consent from the patient to perform a manual BP. Before performing the manual BP, you will need to decide which arm to use. You should avoid using the affected arm if the patient has intravenous fluids in progress or has medical or surgical conditions (e.g. a stroke or breast surgery) that will affect the accuracy of the BP reading as well as cause discomfort to the patient. Check that the patient is rested, and position the patient making sure that the arm is supported by a pillow with the sphygmomanometer placed at the level of the heart (Cork, 2007). Expose the arm by removing any restrictive clothing before placing the correct cuff on the arm. Place the correct-sized cuff around the upper arm, 2–3 cm from the brachial artery, with the tubes facing upright so that there is free access for the stethoscope (BHS, 2009). Figure 4.7(a) shows the most popular position to place the cuff and Figure 4.7(b) shows the correct position for the cuff.

Table 4.2 Blood pressure cuff sizes as recommended by BHS (2009). (British Hypertension Society, 2009).

Size of adult arm	Bladder width and length (cm)	Arm circumference (cm)
Small adult	12×18	<23
Standard adult	12×26	<33
Large adult	12×40	<50

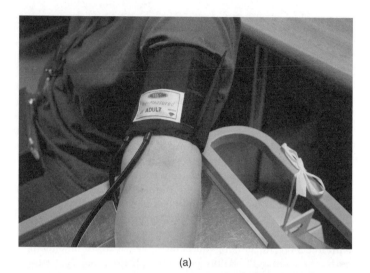

(a)

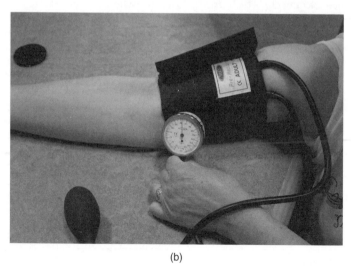

(b)

Fig. 4.7 Blood pressure recording using a sphygmomanometer (photograph).

Place your fingers on the radial pulse and pump up the cuff until the radial pulse can no longer be felt. This occurs because the pressure occludes the blood flow of the radial artery. Observe the dial when you no longer feel the pulse and make a mental note of the level on the sphygmomanometer before deflating the cuff. This gives a baseline to work from to avoid over-inflation of the cuff and discomfort for the patient.

Place the earpieces of the stethoscope in your ears and the chest piece over the brachial pulse. Pump up the cuff to the previous level but then continue to pump a further 30 mmHg (Kozier et al., 2008). Gently deflate the cuff by 2 mmHg at a time until you hear the systolic pressure; a clear tapping sound is heard in time with the heartbeat. This is the first sound you will hear coming in and is the systolic BP. As the cuff deflates further, the sounds become quieter and the last sound heard is the diastolic BP. The sounds that you hear are the Korotkoff's phases. Once you have taken the BP, make sure the patient remains comfortable. Record the systolic and diastolic pressures on the physiological observation chart.

A quick, non-invasive method of assessing blood perfusion is to perform a CRT on the finger of the patient. Lift the finger above the level of the heart and press on the fingertip for 5 seconds (see Fig. 4.8). If there is good perfusion to the fingertip, a pink colour should return to the nail in 2 seconds. If the CRT is prolonged it is a sign of poor perfusion due to systemic vasoconstriction; if it is less than 2 seconds, it is due to systemic vasodilation that is often related to sepsis (Hogston and Marjoram, 2007; CCSI, 2009).

In adults, a normal BP ranges between 100/60 and 140/90 mmHg (NICE, 2006; Doughtery and Lister, 2008). The factors that may affect BP include physical exertion, anxiety, stress, emotional, physiological changes and lifestyle factors. The patient's BP should always be checked under resting conditions (Dougherty and Lister, 2008; Kozier et al., 2008).

Hypertensive (high) BP

If the blood vessels within the body become diseased, for example, as in arteriosclerosis, it may be difficult for blood to flow freely. This can lead to a back flow of blood and therefore increased BP.

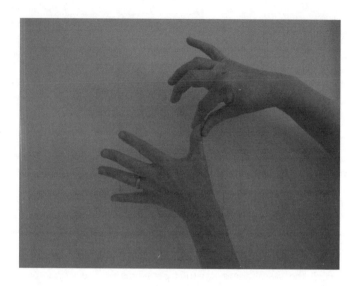

Fig. 4.8 Performing a capillary refill test (photograph).

The body will compensate for a short period of time before the blood vessels become weaker and burst, causing some people to suffer from a cerebral vascular accident (CVA), commonly known as a stroke. A stroke may affect different parts of the brain and may also affect the patient's speech. The patient may show signs of having blurred vision and complain of headaches. The patient may be able to talk to you or be unconscious; the systolic BP may be above 160 mmHg. The World Health Organisation (WHO) defines hypertension as a systolic of 160 mmHg or above and the diastolic of 95 mmHg or above (WHO, 2003; Williams et al., 2004). NICE (2006) recommends that a patient with a persistently raised BP (measured on two separate occasions) above 140/90 is classed as hypertensive. However, if the patient's BP is above 160/100, this is severe hypertension and requires medical intervention. In hypertension, the respiration rate may be faster than normal or slow and shallow. The patient may look flushed because the blood vessels are vasodilated and working hard to pump blood around the body.

Practice point 4.2

A 60-year-old woman has been on holiday in Tenerife and has returned home suffering with diarrhoea and vomiting for 2 days. She is referred by her GP to the Medical Assessment ward. On arrival, her pulse is 125, blood pressure 95/50 and capillary refill is 4 seconds. One hour later, her pulse is 135 and thready, blood pressure is 85/50 and capillary refill time is 6 seconds.

Q1. What do you think is happening to the patient? What action do you need to take?

Q2. From the information read in this chapter and the above case study, what do you think may be happening to the patient using the look, listen and feel approach?

Hypotensive (low) BP and shock

If there is a poor blood volume, this will cause *hypotension* and the heart will try to compensate by beating faster and the blood vessels will constrict (Kozier et al., 2008). When you observe the patient, you may visually notice that their skin looks slightly pale or even cyanosed. This happens because the peripheral blood supply has been diverted to the main organs of the body. The CRT will be delayed (longer than 2 seconds). The patient may be breathing faster because the body is working hard to compensate for the lack of oxygen. When you take the BP and find it to be low with a high pulse rate, your patient is showing signs of *hypovolaemic shock* (Hogston and Marjoram, 2007; CCSI, 2009).

Often, patients may have *hypotension* because the blood vessels have vasodilated (increased in diameter). Blood vessels vasodilate because of messages transmitted from the brain as well as from the influence of medication or disease. If there is a poor supply already, the BP will drop significantly. This means that your patient has developed *neurogenic shock*. The patients will look very pale and may be sweaty and clammy to touch. They may complain of feeling nauseated and dizzy (Hogston and Marjoram, 2007; CCSI, 2009).

Hypotension may also be caused by *septic shock*. The heart will try to compensate by beating faster and you may feel a fast and bounding pulse. The patient may look pink and feel warm to touch or cool and clammy. The CRT may be very fast (less than 2 seconds). Their respiratory rate may initially be fast and shallow and they may also complain of feeling tired or exhausted. The United Kingdom Surviving Sepsis campaign (2007) has produced guidance on how to identify patients with sepsis. Any patient showing any new signs and symptoms of infection (SSI) with two or more of the following observations may be classified as septic: the temperature may be high (above 38°C) or subnormal low (below 36°C); the heart rate will be above 90 bpm; respiratory rate above 20; a change in mental health state; hyperglycaemia (above 6.6 mmol/l) and white cell counts <4 or >12 × 10^9/l (Robson and Daniels, 2008). International guidelines for the management of severe sepsis and septic shock were published in 2008 (Dellinger et al., 2008).

Practice point 4.3

Access the surviving sepsis campaign website:
www.survivingsepsis.org

Think of a patient you may have cared for who was septic and compare the care management against the National Guidance on identifying, assessing and managing a septic patient.

Sometimes the heart muscle is damaged and cannot pump as efficiently. This damage can be the result of a heart attack or because some parts of the heart are not working because of cardiac arrhythmias due to an imbalance in urea and electrolytes. You may have difficulty in feeling the radial pulse because of peripheral shutdown, or the pulse maybe irregular because of abnormal heart rhythms. The CRT will be delayed and the BP will be low. This means that the heart is unable to pump sufficient blood through the body, and this leads to poor blood supply to the organs and is known as *cardiogenic shock* (Hogston and Marjoram, 2007).

The final type of shock that affects the BP is *anaphylactic shock*. This may be caused by a reaction to bee stings, food (e.g. peanuts and shell fish) or even medication. The highest anaphylactic risk in adult healthcare settings is from blood transfusions. In anaphylactic shock, the respiratory rate will be increased, the pulse will be bounding with a CRT less than 2 seconds and the BP will be low. The patient's skin may also feel flushed, hot and sweaty (Resuscitation Council UK, 2006). Anaphylactic shock is a medical emergency. If you observe any of the above signs of shock in the patient, you must call for senior help – for example, the outreach team or medical emergency team or call 999 immediately.

Electrocardiograph
If the patient has an abnormal rhythm and irregular pulse, it may be advisable to order or perform an electrocardiograph (ECG). This is a non-invasive method of measuring the electrical activity of the heart and is used in line with other methods of cardiovascular assessments.

Look, listen and feel
To be able to assess a patient's CVS correctly and accurately, a systematic approach needs to be adopted using 'Look, Listen and Feel'.

Look at the patient's skin colour assessing whether it is pale, grey, flushed or cyanosed. Look for any signs of perspiration, which may indicate signs of shock and also look for signs of peripheral cyanosis, which may indicate a poor circulating volume. Listen to the patient's Korotkoff's sounds when performing a manual BP. Listen for alarms that may arise from alterations in the patient's parameters. Feel and check manually for pulse even when using electronic BP devices to assess the rate and character of the pulse. Feel the patient's skin – is it cold, clammy, warm to touch or how sweaty does the skin feel? Finally, look at the vital signs chart and compare all previous trends in BP, pulse and MAP.

CONCLUSION
In this chapter, we have discussed the anatomy and physiology of the CVS – a knowledge of the heart and circulation will assist you in performing a cardiovascular assessment competently. Throughout this chapter, we have discussed the importance of using the correct equipment and reiterated that healthcare professionals must be competent to perform a BP, pulse and capillary refill test.

Observing and recording of the pulse rate, rhythm and regulatory, BP, capillary refill and using the look, listen and feel approach will provide a comprehensive assessment. There is a wide range of factors that may affect the cardiovascular status of the patient, which will inform the individual assessment. It is essential to inform and gain consent from the patient prior to performing physiological observations. It is also necessary to follow infection prevention procedures and document accurate recordings.

REFERENCES

Bellamy JE, Pugh H, and Sanders DJ (2008). The trouble with blood pressure cuffs. *British Medical Journal* **337**, 515–516.

British Hypertension Society (2009). *Blood Pressure Measurement BHS* www.bhsoc.org [Accessed 12th October 2009].

Cork A (2007). Theory and practice of manual blood pressure measurement. *Nursing Standard* **22**(14), 14–16.

Critical Care Skills Institute (CCSI) (2009). *Acute Illness Management. AIM Course Manual.* Greater Manchester, Critical Care Skills Institute. www.gmcriticalcareskillsinstitute.org.uk.

Davey P (2008). *ECG at a Glance.* Oxford, Wiley-Blackwell.

Dellinger RP, Levy MM, Carlet JM, et al. (2008). Surviving sepsis campaign: International guidelines for management of severe sepsis and septic shock: 2008. *Intensive Care Medicine* **34**, 17–10.

Department of Health (2009). *Competencies for Recognising and Responding to Acutely Ill Patients in Hospital.* http://www.dh.gov.uk/publications. [Accessed 12th March 2010].

Dougherty L and Lister S (2008). *The Royal Marsden Hospital Manual of Clinical Nursing Procedures.* 7th edn. Oxford, Wiley-Blackwell.

Hasan MA, Thomas TA, and Prys-Robert C (1993). Comparison of automatic oscillometric arterial pressure measurement with conventional auscultatory measurement in labour ward. *British Journal of Anaesthesia* **70**(2), 141–144.

Hogston R and Marjoram BA (2007). *Foundations of Nursing Practice.* 3rd edn. Hampshire, Palgrave.

Kozier B, Erb G, Berman A, Snyder S, Lake R, and Harvey S (2008). *Fundamentals of Nursing, Concepts, Process and Practice.* Essex, Pearson Education.

Marieb EN (2009). *Essentials of Human Anatomy and Physiology* 9th edn. San Francisco, Pearson Benjamin Cummings.

Medicines and Health products Regulatory Agency (MHRA) (2001). *Tissue Necrosis Caused by Pulse Oximeter Probes.* SN2001 (08). http://www.mhra.gov.uk/index.htm.

Montague SE, Watson R, Herbert R (2005). *Physiology for Nursing Practice* 3rd ed. Oxford, Bailliere Tindall.

National Institute for Health and Clinical Excellence (NICE) (2006). *Hypertension: Management of Hypertension in Adults in Primary Care.* NICE clinical guideline 34. London, NICE.

National Institute for Health and Clinical Excellence (NICE) (2007). *Acutely Ill Patients in Hospital: Recognition of and Response to Acute Illness in Adults in Hospital.* NICE clinical guideline 50. London, NICE.

National Patient Safety Agency (NPSA) (2007). *Recognising and Responding Appropriately to Early Signs of Deterioration in Hospitalised Patients.* www.nspa.nhs.uk [Accessed 17th February 2009].

O'Brien E, Waeber B, Parati G, Staessen J, and Myers MG (2001). Blood pressure measuring devices: recommendations of the European Society of Hypertension. *British Medical Journal* **322**, 531–536; doi:10.1136/bmj.322.7285.531.

Resuscitation Council UK (2006). *Advanced Life Support.* 5th edn. London, Resuscitation Council UK.

Robson W and Daniels R (2008). The Sepsis six: helping patients to survive sepsis. *British Journal of Nursing* **17**(1), 16–21.

Sadik R, Walker C, and Elliott D (2007). Respiration and circulation. In: *Foundations of Nursing Practice Leading the Way*, Hogston R and Marjoram BA (eds). London, Palgrave Macmillan.

Sharman J (2007). Clinical skills: cardiac rhythm recognition and monitoring. *British Journal of Nursing* **16**(5), 306–311.

Thornett A (2007). New skills for HCAs: taking a blood pressure. *British Journal of Health Care Assistants* **1**(3), 133–135.

Tortora G and Derrickson B (2006). *Principles of Anatomy and Physiology.* 11th edn. USA, John Wiley and Sons Inc.

Tortora GJ and Nielsen MT (2009). *Principles of Human Anatomy.* 11th edn. USA, John Wiley and Sons Inc.

Walsh M and Crumbie A (eds) (2007). Caring for the patient with a cardiovascular disorder. In: *Watson's Clinical Nursing and Related Sciences.* 7th edn. London, Balliere Tindall Elsevier.

Waugh A and Grant A (2001). *Ross and Wilson Anatomy and Physiology in Health and Illness.* 9th edn. London, Churchill Livingstone.

Williams B, Poulter NR, Brown MJ, et al. (2004). The BHS guidelines Working Party Guidelines for management of hypertension: Report of the Fourth Working Party of the British Hypertension Society. *Journal of Human Hypertension* **18**(3), 139–185.

Woods S, Froelicher E, and Motzer S (2000). *Cardiac Nursing.* 4th edn. Philadelphia, Lippincott.

World Health Organisation (WHO) (2003). International Society of Hypertension (ISH) statement on management of hypertension. *Journal of Hypertension* **21**, 1983–1992.

Temperature

5

INTRODUCTION

Temperature is a significant component of the patients' physiological observations and has been called 'the forgotten vital sign' (Smith et al., 2005). It is a useful indicator in the assessment of any new infection or ongoing illness (Mains et al., 2008). Measuring the body temperature will provide information on how hot or cold the body is in relation to the amount of heat (energy) being used. Chemical reactions that take place in the body to create energy for the cells are known as *metabolism* (Waugh and Grant, 2001).

Metabolism is the total amount of chemical changes that occur within the body to convert food into fuel. The body requires a constant temperature of around 36.0–37.5°C to maintain metabolism (Dougherty and Lister, 2008). More recently, normal adult body temperature has been defined as 36.5–37.5°C (National Institute for Clinical Excellence (NICE), 2008). A by-product of metabolism is heat, which can be measured using a thermometer. If the temperature is high, it is an indication that the metabolic rate is faster than normal and also that the body has an increased need for fuel to feed the tissues, in the form of oxygen and glucose. If the temperature is low, it indicates that metabolism is slowing down.

LEARNING OUTCOMES

By the end of this chapter, you will be able to discuss the following:

❏ The role of thermoregulation within the body
❏ What factors influence temperature

Vital Signs for Nurses: An Introduction to Clinical Observations, First Edition.
Joyce Smith and Rachel Roberts.

❏ What is the normal/abnormal range for temperature
❏ How to perform a temperature measurement

THE ROLE OF THERMOREGULATION WITHIN THE BODY

During illness, the body will experience changes within the physiological state, such as an increase in the respiratory rate, pulse rate and temperature. These changes are controlled by an area in the brain known as the *hypothalamus* (Roberts, 2008). The hypothalamus regulates the temperature of the organs, tissues and circulating blood and acts like a thermostat found within a central heating system (Broom, 2007; Roberts, 2008). The dial of the thermostat can be set to whatever temperature range you wish. In the body's case, the hypothalamus sets its thermostat to run at a core temperature of 37°C because human beings are 'homoiothermic' (Fulbrook, 1993; Waugh and Grant, 2006) and function at their best within this range. However, in times of infection, the hypothalamus may reset the thermostat and allow the body temperature to rise in order to create a fever.

Fever has been defined as 'an elevation of body temperature above the normal daily variation' (NICE, 2007, p. 17). The fever will increase the metabolic rate for the body to fight off the illness or infection (Broom, 2007; Roberts, 2008) and also hinder the growth of invading viral or bacterial micro-organisms (Glasper and Richardson, 2006). This increase in the metabolic rate will consequently increase the amount of extra glucose and oxygen required by the body. For further information, please refer to Chapter 10 regarding nutrition.

When the hypothalamus resets the thermostat to a temperature above 37°C, the body then triggers physiological mechanisms to create more heat by causing the body to start shivering and develop goose bumps on the skin. The patient may complain of feeling cold and hungry, as the body sends messages that it needs more fuel to fight the infection (Mains et al., 2008). The body also relies on human behaviour to help it control the body temperature. Feeling cold and shivery may cause the patient to want to put on extra clothing or bedding to maintain the body temperature (Mains et al., 2008).

Another mechanism used to control thermoregulation is the brain's ability to control the size of the diameters of the blood vessels, causing them to either vasodilate or constrict. A higher temperature will trigger the body to release a hormone called *adrenaline*. Adrenaline will act on the heart to make it beat faster and therefore increase the pulse rate. It will also act on the peripheral blood vessels and cause them to vasoconstrict. This action means that the blood can remain as close to the core of the body and away from the surface of the skin, which in turn reduces the amount of heat loss (Roberts, 2008).

As we have discussed previously, body temperature is a measure of the body's ability to produce and get rid of heat; it represents the balance of the metabolic processes taking place within the human body (Dougherty and Lister, 2008) and helps to maintain homeostasis. The body is very good at regulating its temperature within a narrow, safe range in spite of large variations in temperature outside the body. To create heat, the body relies on the metabolic activities of the major organs. Some illnesses and diseases can also impact on the range of body temperature – for example, a damaged liver, which in normal health produces lots of heat and energy, will be less efficient and so the body will function at a cooler body temperature.

To release heat, the body uses the skin and sweat glands to cool the body down through processes called *convection* and *conduction* (Tortora and Derrickson, 2006; Dougherty and Lister, 2008). In fact, up to 60% of the body's heat can be lost through the head if left uncovered (Cooper, 2006).

NORMAL BODY TEMPERATURE

Normal body temperature in health remains constant around 36.8°C, although this can range in adults between 36.5 and 37.5°C (NICE, 2008). The temperature will fluctuate throughout the day (between 0.5°C and 1.5°C) and will be influenced by activities such as exercise, eating, ovulation in women and the body's circadian rhythms. The temperature can be measured in either Celsius (°C) or Fahrenheit (°F). Most people believe that the 'normal' body temperature is 36°C or 98.6°F, but this is an average of normal body temperature.

WHAT FACTORS INFLUENCE BODY TEMPERATURE?

There are environmental factors that will influence the body temperature such as which hemisphere you live in. If you live in the tropics, you will be used to hot weather, but if you live at the North Pole, your body will be used to cold weather. The weather and seasons do affect what clothing choices people make to maintain their body temperature. Physiological ageing also affects the efficiency of the body and its ability to regulate body temperature, including chronic or acute diseases. Medications that patients take may also affect the body's ability to regulate their body temperature (Dougherty and Lister, 2008).

DEFINING FEVER (PYREXIA)

Fever is the body's response to an invading micro-organism and is therefore a useful clinical indication of the immune system fighting off an infection (Broom, 2007). However, individuals have their own internally set thermostat, and therefore, NICE (2007) has published a broad definition of 'an elevation of body temperature above the normal daily variation'. Patients should be treated as unique individuals and therefore their unique body temperature range should also be recognised. For some patients, normal body thermostat averages at 36.4–36.5°C, so when they become unwell and their temperature rises to 37.2°C, they complain of feeling very poorly. However, within the hospital setting, a temperature reading of 37.2°C may not have been taken into consideration as being higher than normal for the patient and may be accepted by nursing staff as normal. Therefore, when assessing temperature, it may be useful to find out from the patient whether they know what their average body temperature is when they are well. There are different graded definitions for temperature ranges that have been collated in Table 5.1.

A LOW BODY TEMPERATURE – HYPOTHERMIA

If the thermostat of the body is unable to maintain the body temperature within a normal range, the body's core temperature will begin to cool down (Kemp, 2008). Hypothermia is associated with ageing and exposure to a cold environment (Kemp, 2008). As you can see in Table 5.1, NICE (2008) defines hypothermia as a core temperature <36°C. Studies have found that as much as 90% of surgical patients will experience hypothermia preoperatively (Neno, 2005; Cooper, 2006).

Table 5.1 Temperature ranges.

Definition	Temperature range (°C)	Source
Hyperpyrexia	>40.0	Dougherty and Lister (2008)
Moderate to high pyrexia	38.0–40.0	Dougherty and Lister (2008)
Low grade pyrexia	36.7–38.0	Dougherty and Lister (2008)
Comfortable, warm pre and postoperatively	36.5–37.5	NICE (2008)
Normothermic	36.0–36.5	Dougherty and Lister (2008)
Hypothermia	Core <36	NICE (2008)
Mild hypothermia	32–35	Resuscitation Council UK (2006)
Moderate hypothermia	30–32	Resuscitation Council UK (2006)
Severe hypothermia	<30	Resuscitation Council UK (2006)

An abnormal low body temperature can be very serious, even life threatening (Resuscitation Council, 2006). Low body temperature may occur from exposure to the cold, shock states, alcohol or drug use or in certain metabolic disorders such as diabetes or hypothyroidism. A low body temperature may also be present with an infection, particularly in older adults or people who are frail. An overwhelming infection, such as sepsis, may also cause an abnormally low body temperature (Smith et al., 2005; Kemp, 2008). Recognition and treatment of hypothermia is essential because it can become a medical emergency (Smith et al., 2005; Resuscitation Council, 2006; Kemp, 2008).

A HIGH BODY TEMPERATURE – HYPERTHERMIA

Hyperthermia will occur when the body is no longer able to control its own thermostat, causing it to absorb too much heat at a faster rate than it can cool itself down, which in turn starts to damage the cells of the body. An example of this is heat stroke. Heat stroke occurs when the body fails to regulate its own temperature and the body temperature continues to rise. Symptoms of heat stroke include alteration in mental abilities such as confusion, delirium or unconsciousness and may present similar symptoms as septic shock. The skin may look flushed and red and may be hot to touch or alternatively dry and oedematous (Resuscitation Council, 2006).

Practice point 5.1

While bed bathing a 60-year-old post-op laparotomy patient, you observe that the patient's skin looks bright red around the wound dressing and is tracking down the abdomen. The tympanic temperature is 38.5°C; respiratory rate has increased to 28; BP is 110/70 and pulse is 125. The patient is complaining of pain around his wound site.

What do you think is happening to the patient and what action will you take to prevent further deterioration?

Failure of the body's thermostat in the hyperthermic patient can lead to life-threatening conditions. Temperatures of 41°C can induce fitting, which is sometimes called *febrile convulsions*. Temperatures between 41 and 43°C will cause damage to the cells in the brain, and this can result in brain damage or even death (Mains et al., 2008). Certain types of medicines such as antibiotics, painkillers and antihistamines can bring on a 'drug fever'. For example, if you are going on a holiday abroad and require certain vaccinations, you may have side effects that will increase the body temperature.

The reasons to take a body temperature

A patient's body temperature is measured to

- detect a fever;
- detect abnormally low body temperature (hypothermia) in people who have been exposed to cold;
- detect abnormally high body temperature (hyperthermia) in people who have been exposed to heat;
- detect hyperpyrexia (high temperature), which can result in the death of cells within the body and can be life threatening;
- help monitor the effectiveness of drugs used to reduce a fever – for example, paracetamol;
- help plan for pregnancy by determining whether a woman is ovulating.

Where is the body temperature measured?

There are a variety of manufacturers who produce thermometers, all of which have benefits and disadvantages (Roberts, 2008).

Body temperature can be measured in many locations of the body such as

- the forehead;
- the ear (tympanic);
- the armpit (axilla);
- the mouth (oral).

The preferred route for taking a temperature is non-invasive using a disposable thermometer, and NICE (2007) supports the use of both tympanic and disposable chemical dot thermometers, whereas the use of the rectal thermometers is not recommended because it potentially can cause harm to the rectum and is not socially acceptable, despite providing an accurate method of ascertaining the core temperature of the body (O'Toole, 1998; Farley and McLafferty, 2008). Thermometers require maintenance and servicing and this should be completed in conjunction with manufacturers' recommendations.

Forehead (temporal) thermometer

One method of taking a temporal temperature is to press the soft discs against the forehead and hold the thermometer in place for the required amount of time until the reading is displayed. Other types include plastic strips with numbers that are placed against the forehead and the temperature makes the numbers change colour or light up. Clean and dispose of the thermometer as per manufacturers' guidelines or per trust policy and document the temperature on the physiological observation chart. These thermometers are not as accurate as the electronic or ear thermometers.

Disposable thermometers

Disposable thermometers are thin flat pieces of plastic with colour dots and temperature markings on one end (Fig. 5.1). The colour of the dots shows the temperature. Disposable thermometers can be used in the mouth or axilla. These thermometers are safe and accurate and do not contain glass, latex or mercury.

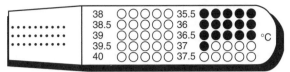

This example reads 37.0°C.

Fig. 5.1 Disposable thermometer.

Ear thermometers (tympanic)

There are different manufacturers' models that use infrared light to measure body temperature. The small cone-shaped end of the thermometer has a disposable cover for infection prevention and is placed inside the ear and held in place until the body temperature is shown on the digital display, with results appearing in 2 seconds. Tympanic thermometers are popular in adult care settings (NICE, 2007; Mains et al., 2008; Fig. 5.2).

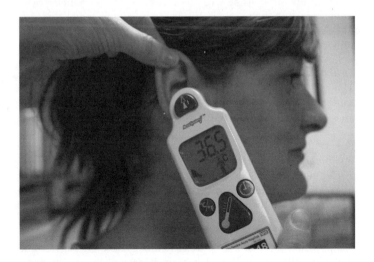

Fig. 5.2 A tympanic thermometer (photograph).

When using tympanic thermometers, ensure that the disposable probe is of the correct size for the ear canal. Explain to the patient what you are about to do and obtain their consent. Then gently pull the pinna (top of the ear) backwards so that the ear canal will be straightened and gently insert the thermometer until the ear canal is sealed. Once an accurate position is obtained, press the button on the tympanic thermometer and wait for it to beep. Gently remove the temperature probe from the ear canal and read the display screen to obtain the temperature. If not, repeat the process again. Once the reading is obtained, discard the disposable cover in the clinical waste bin. Ear wax or ear infections should not affect the accuracy of the reading. Ideally, patients should have their own dedicated tympanic thermometer to reduce infection risks to others (Mains et al., 2008).

Electronic thermometers
Electronic thermometers are made of plastic and shaped like a pencil, with a display window at one end and a temperature probe at the other. They work by measuring how well electricity travels through the wire. Electronic thermometers may be used in the mouth, armpit and rectum, but a risk assessment should be undertaken while deciding the most appropriate route.

Oral temperature
The oral route used to be popular, but this has been replaced by safer non-invasive methods (NICE, 2007; Mains et al., 2008). To get an accurate temperature, the person must be able to breathe through the nose and not be at risk of fitting or biting on the thermometer. Ensure that you perform a risk assessment that the oral route for obtaining the temperature is indeed the most appropriate method.

Having obtained the patient's consent, position the digital or disposable thermometer under the tongue, just to one side of the centre and close the lips tightly around it. Leave the thermometer in place for the required amount of time, as suggested by the manufacturers. Some digital thermometers give a series of short bleeps when the reading is done. Remove the thermometer and document the temperature. Clean or dispose of the thermometer as per manufacturers' guidelines or per trust policy. Reassure your patient and make sure they are comfortable.

How to take an armpit (axilla) temperature?
Digital or chemical dot thermometers (Fig. 5.1) can be used in the axilla and are useful in obtaining a temperature when other routes are not available, but the thermometer must stay in the axilla for 3 minutes and its accuracy has not always been reliable (Perry and Potter, 2002; Roberts, 2008). Armpit temperature readings maybe as much as 0.6–1°C lower than an oral temperature reading.

TEMPERATURE ASSESSMENT USING LOOK, LISTEN AND FEEL

Look at the patients and talk to them to find out if they are able to maintain their own airway. Listen to what the patients tell you and find out how they are feeling. The patients may tell you that they are feeling shivery and sometimes hot and at other times cold. This is also a sign that there are changes in temperature. Look at the colour of the skin; is it pale, cyanosed, pink or flushed? Is the skin burnt or bruised? Does the skin feel hot to touch? It may be an early sign of infection or dehydration. If pulse oximetry is available, record the patient's oxygen saturation (SpO_2). It may be difficult to obtain if the patient is hypothermic. Call for senior help if you have not done so already and consider the use of oxygen therapy. Assess the circulation by looking at the colour of the patient and perform capillary refill time (CRT) as well as by feeling for a manual pulse. A patient with fever will lose heat and sweat out fluid, becoming dehydrated. The CRT will be prolonged in a dehydrated patient and the pulse will feel weak and the peripheries such as hands and feet will be cool. Inform a senior member of the clinical team of your clinical findings.

Listen for any noisy breathing that may indicate an airway obstruction. If the patient is unresponsive, call for senior nursing and medical help at once and put them in the recovery position. If the patient has a febrile convulsion, maintain the patient's airway safety as much as is reasonably practicable and call for urgent assistance. Assess the level of decreased consciousness, and if the patient is only responsive to pain or is unresponsive, call for help and protect the airway in line with basic life support principles.

Feel the patient's skin and assess whether it feels hot, sweaty or clammy. The patient may feel pain on touch – for example, in patients with arthritis – so be gentle and maintain their dignity. Report the information you gather to the nurse in charge once you have taken the temperature and completed all the other physiological observations.

Practice point 5.2

A 72-year-old gentleman has been gardening all day on a hot summer's day. His grandchild happens to be a nurse and she comes to visit him. The gentleman complains to her that he is feeling sick and has got a headache.

Using the look, listen and feel approach, what should the nurse do?

TEMPERATURE MANAGEMENT

The two main areas of temperature management will be when the patient has either hypothermia or hyperthermia and the interventions provided will be dependent on the healthcare environment.

The development of hypothermia is usually accidental or unintentional – for example, when an elderly person falls at home and is unable to get up again. There is an increased risk of hypothermia where there is drug or alcohol intake, illness, injury or neglect (Resuscitation Council, 2006). To prevent the onset of hypothermia, patients can be educated about how to take preventative measures such as keeping their house warm, wearing enough warm and dry clothing and having a hot meal with plenty of warm, non-alcoholic drinks.

It has been recognised that preoperative education about prevention of hypothermia will be beneficial to the patient (NICE, 2008). The document on management of inadvertent perioperative hypothermia in adults, *Clinical guideline 65*, NICE (2008), recommends that patients, families and carers should be informed that keeping warm will reduce the risk of postoperative complications and that patients should bring in extra supplies of warm clothing such as a dressing gown, socks and slippers to help them maintain their body heat. The document also recommends that healthcare staff be trained in the use of warming devices in conjunction with infection prevention policies. The patient should arrive to theatre and have the temperature recorded before being anaesthetised and it should be above 36.0°C. The document outlines the parameters for temperature regulation intraoperatively and postoperatively (NICE, 2008).

The method of rewarming does depend on the degree of hypothermia and is divided into three areas – passive warming, active warming and active core warming (Farley and McLafferty, 2008). Passive warming would be appropriate for patients with mild hypothermia and involves simple, practical measures of removing wet and cold clothing, drying the patient and replacing clothing with warmed clothes and prewarmed blankets. The head should be covered with a hat or head covering to retain heat, as up to 60% of heat can be lost from the head (Cooper, 2006). Active warming is most appropriate for patients with moderate-to-severe hypothermia. If the patient is able to get into a hot bath, this will assist in raising the body temperature as well as the use of warming blankets (Farley and Mc Lafferty, 2008). Active core warming relates to patients with a core temperature <32°C with the purpose of avoiding cardiac arrest. Senior medical and nursing intervention will be required. If the patient is still breathing, the senior medical staff will require warmed (40–46°C) and humidified oxygen as well as warmed intravenous fluids. Warming techniques that can be accessed in the acute hospital setting include peritoneal and bladder lavage; haemofiltration or dialysis may be considered (Resuscitation Council, 2006). The temperature should be measured and monitored frequently during the rewarming process and different authors recommend different rates for rewarming from 1–2°C to 0.3–1.2°C per hour (Farley and McLafferty, 2008). It must be remembered that as the body warms, the metabolic rate will rise and this will increase demand for more oxygen and glucose to sustain it; so the body does need to adapt and warm up slowly to respond to the changes in the metabolic rate and the temperature.

Supportive management of hyperthermia includes the use of medications such as paracetamol and ibrufen. These help promote comfort but will not prevent febrile convulsions and so should not be used specifically for this (NICE, 2007). It must be remembered that the body raises the temperature in order to allow the immune system to fight more efficiently (Broom, 2007). The use of tepid sponging and the use of fans are not of any medical benefit and will provide comfort only. There are a variety of blankets on the market that can be used to warm or cool body temperature, and within critical care, there is the development of therapeutic hypothermia in post-cardiac arrest patients (Resuscitation Council, 2006; Kemp, 2008). Simple measures such as drinking plenty of fluid to rehydrate and eating to fuel up the body to fight the infection are also essential in the management of hyperthermia.

CONCLUSION

In this chapter, we have briefly discussed the role of the hypothalamus in temperature regulation. Measuring the temperature is one of the vital physiological observations required in monitoring and managing adult patients (NICE, 2007). A basic knowledge of how the temperature is regulated and the factors that influence thermoregulation aids in performing a temperature assessment competently. There are different thermometers available to measure temperature and the healthcare professional must assess the patient for use of the most appropriate device. Hypothermia and hyperthermia may affect patients in any environment. The accurate recording of the patients' temperature not only alerts the nurse to early signs of infection and illness but also ensures that patients are treated in a timely manner.

Throughout this chapter, we have discussed the importance of using the correct equipment and reiterated that healthcare professionals must be competent to monitor and record temperature. Observing and recording of temperature using the look, listen and feel approach will provide a comprehensive assessment. It is essential to inform and gain consent from the patient prior to performing the procedure. It is also necessary to follow infection prevention procedures and document accurate recordings.

REFERENCES

Broom M (2007). Physiology of fever. *Paediatric Nursing* **19**(6), 40–45.
Cooper S (2006). The effect of preoperative warming on patients' postoperative temperatures. *AORN Journal* **82**(50), 1074–1088.
Dougherty L and Lister S (2008). *The Royal Marsden Hospital Manual of Clinical Nursing Procedures*. 7th edn. Oxford, Wiley-Blackwell.

Farley A and McLafferty E (2008). Nursing management of the patient with hypothermia. *Nursing Standard* **22**(917), 43–46.

Fulbrook P (1993). Core temperature measurement in adults: a literature review. *Journal of Advanced Nursing* **18**(9), 1451–1460.

Glasper A and Richardson J (2006). *A Textbook of Children and Young People's Nursing*. Edinburgh, Churchill Livingstone.

Kemp P (2008). Hypothermia: causes and management. *British Journal of Healthcare Assistants* **2**(12), 586–588.

Mains J, Coxall K, and Lloyd H (2008). Measuring temperature. *Nursing Standard* **22**(29), 44–47.

National Institute for Clinical Excellence (NICE) (2007). *Feverish Illness: Assessment and Initial Management in Children Younger than Five Years of Age*. Clinical guideline 47. London, NICE.

Neno R (2005). Hypothermia: assessment treatment and prevention. *Nursing Standard* **19**(20), 47–54.

NICE (2008). *Inadvertent Perioperative Hypothermia. The Management of Inadvertent Perioperative Hypothermia in Adults*. Clinical guideline 65. London, NICE.

O'Toole S (1998). Temperature measurement devices. *Professional Nurse.* **13**(11), 779–786.

Perry P and Potter P (2002). *Clinical Nursing Skills and Techniques*. 5th edn. St Louis, MO, Mosby.

Resuscitation Council UK (2006). *Advanced Life Support*. 5th edn. London, Resuscitation Council (UK).

Roberts S (2008). Paediatrics: caring for a child with a temperature. *British Journal of Healthcare Assistants* **2**(7), 327–329.

Smith J, Bland S, and Mullett S (2005). Temperature – the forgotten vital sign. *Accident and Emergency Nursing* **13**, 247–250.

Tortora G and Derrickson B (2006). *Principles of Anatomy and Physiology*. 11th edn. USA, John Wiley and Sons Inc.

Waugh A and Grant A (2001). *Ross and Wilson Anatomy and Physiology in Health and Illness*. 9th edn. London, Churchill Livingstone.

Waugh A and Grant A (2006). *Ross and Wilson Anatomy and Physiology in Health and Illness*. 10th edn. London, Churchill Livingstone.

Urine Output

6

INTRODUCTION

The kidneys are the organs that process and purify the internal fluids within the body. They have been described as the equivalent of a sanitation plant that processes and purifies waste to make the water supply drinkable. The role and purpose of sanitation processing plants are often unappreciated by local towns and their population until they break down – much like the kidney in human beings (Marieb, 2009).

Urine is a waste product that is produced by the kidneys. The kidneys are important in controlling the body's fluid balance. Checking the urine output of patients when undertaking physiological observations is a simple and effective way to find out how the kidneys function and thereby the hydration status of a patient. Poor management of urine output can lead to acute kidney injury (AKI), also previously known as acute renal failure (ARF) (Davies, 2009). AKI recognition has been found to be poorly recognised (National Confidential Enquiry into Patient Outcome and Death (NCEPOD), 2009).

LEARNING OUTCOMES

By the end of this chapter, you will be able to discuss the following:

❑ The function of the kidneys within the body
❑ Factors that influence urine output
❑ The normal–abnormal range for urine output

Vital Signs for Nurses: An Introduction to Clinical Observations, First Edition.
Joyce Smith and Rachel Roberts.
© 2011 Joyce Smith and Rachel Roberts. Published 2011 by Blackwell Publishing Ltd.

❏ How to measure urine output and fluid balance accurately
❏ How to obtain urine sampling and testing
❏ Renal case scenario

THE ANATOMY AND PHYSIOLOGY OF THE KIDNEYS

The kidneys are two bean-shaped organs that are found situated behind the abdomen. Each adult kidney is approximately 11 cm long, 6 cm wide and 3 cm thick and weighs 150 g (Fillingham and Douglas, 2004). They are found in the abdominal cavity and lie posterior to the parietal peritoneum within the retroperitoneal space. The right kidney is lower than the left kidney because of the position of the liver. To add protection and warmth, the kidneys are covered in a layer of fat that has a cushioning effect. The kidneys produce urine, which is then sent via the ureters to the bladder. The bladder drains the urine into the *urethra* and a person then goes to the toilet to *urinate* (Waugh and Grant, 2001).

The outer layer of the kidney is a strong, fibrous layer. This layer protects the renal cortex and the renal pyramids, also known as the *medulla*. The cortex contains the filtration unit of the kidneys, which are known as *glomerular filtration capsules*. Urine is formed in the glomerulus through a process known as *filtration*. The glomerulus is part of the *nephron* (O'Callaghan and Brenner, 2001).

Several complex processes occur within the nephron that include filtration, *reabsorption* and *secretion*. The kidney maintains the balance of water and electrolytes within the body through this process. Put simply, the kidney responds to changes in the body to retain salts (e.g. sodium and potassium) and water. When healthy, the kidney ensures that the right amount of water, sodium, potassium, calcium, magnesium and many more substances are kept at the correct level to maintain the body's acid–base balance (O'Callaghan and Brenner, 2001).

The kidney is also influenced by powerful hormones in regulating the fluid balance of the body. These four hormones are called antidiuretic hormone (ADH), aldosterone, atrial natriuretic peptide (ANP) and parathyroid hormone. The kidney also produces hormones for the body. These are renin, vitamin D, erythropoietin and prostaglandins. The kidney is supported by a vast blood supply made up of millions of capillaries, and the capillaries are

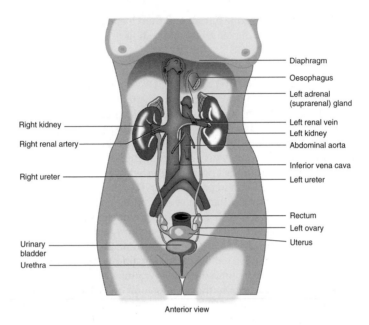

Right kidney

Right renal artery

Right ureter

Urinary
bladder

Urethra

Diaphragm

Oesophagus

Left adrenal
(suprarenal) gland

Left renal vein

Left kidney

Abdominal aorta

Inferior vena cava

Left ureter

Rectum

Left ovary

Uterus

Anterior view

Fig. 6.1 Organs of the urinary system in a female. Tortora and Derrickson, 2006; reprinted with permission from John Wiley and Sons Inc.

influenced by changes in pressures (O'Callaghan and Brenner, 2001) (see Fig. 6.1).

THE ROLE AND FUNCTION OF THE KIDNEYS WITHIN THE BODY

The kidneys are organs that maintain the balance of fluid within the body. This is known as *homeostasis*. This means that all the compartments in the body are kept within normal ranges. These compartments contain water and salts, commonly known as *electrolytes*.

The main functions of the kidneys are as follows:

- Filtering the blood to remove waste products of metabolism such as urea and creatinine

- Controlling fluid and circulating volume status, that is, fluid balance
- Regulating the electrolytes in the blood
- Keeping the blood acid–base balance within a normal range
- Controlling blood pressure using the renin–angiotensin mechanism
- Producing erythropoietin
- Controlling the reabsorption of calcium and vitamin D

When healthy, the kidney requires a large amount of the blood supply to provide it with significant amounts of oxygen just to perform its normal function. The kidney's blood supply comes from the aorta and the inferior vena cava. The kidney is such a complex, busy processing unit that it needs to use around 25% of the oxygen supplied in the blood, which is equivalent to the kidney using a quarter of the body's cardiac output. So, not only do the kidneys require care and high maintenance but they also need plenty of blood supply with the blood vessels well filled in order to filter and produce urine.

The kidneys become particularly at risk to harm and developing AKI when there is either lack of oxygen or poor blood supply. Lack of both oxygen and blood supply may be catastrophic for the kidney. This is because a poor blood supply will lead to low flow of blood through the kidneys. A drop in blood flow leads to a drop in pressure in the kidneys and this leads to *poor perfusion* of the kidney. If the kidney is poorly perfused, it will stop functioning properly and this may lead to renal failure (Adam and Osborne, 2001; Perkins and Kisiel, 2005; Critical Care Skills Institute (CCSI), 2009).

Regulation of blood pressure (BP)

Blood pressure (BP) is controlled through a complex system known as *autoregulation*. BP is the pressure exerted on the arterial walls by the volume of blood ejected from the heart. The peak pressure is called *systolic pressure* and the minimum value is the *diastolic pressure*. The mean arterial pressure (MAP) is the average pressure exerted via the cardiac cycle and is directly related to vital organ perfusion. The normal range of MAP is 70–105 mmHg. Most electronic BP machines will calculate the MAP (CCSI, 2009). There are several ways to calculate the MAP but here is one way to do it. To calculate the MAP,

$$\text{MAP} = \text{Diastolic} + \frac{(\text{systolic} - \text{diastolic})}{3}$$

Practice point 6.1

The nurse-in-charge asked you to take a manual BP from a post-operative patient. The BP is 120/60. The doctor has requested that the MAP should be maintained above 70 mmHg. Calculate the MAP using the formula above.

The kidneys require good perfusion pressures to function. As a general rule, most kidneys will function when the *MAP is 65 mmHg* or above. However, in renal and hypertensive disease, this figure may be higher. If the MAP drops below 65 mmHg, then the kidneys will not have the pressure and blood supply they need to function and may stop working and cause renal failure (CCSI, 2009).

Maintaining fluid balance of the body

To make a skilled fluid balance review on a patient, you need to have an understanding of the principles of the fluid compartments within the body and how they function.

Essentially, an average 70-kg human male is 42 l of fluid covered in skin. The 42 l is divided into different fluid compartments. The two main fluid compartments are called the *intracellular* (inside the cells) and *extracellular* (outside the cells) compartments. The extracellular space is subdivided into the *vascular* (blood vessels) and *interstitial* (space between the cells and the blood vessels) compartments. Water, electrolytes and nutrients are dissolved in the blood and can travel between compartments via a semiperme-able membrane (sieve-like layer; Fig. 6.2). The movement of fluid is achieved through the process of osmosis, which is a passive process (Jenkins et al., 2010).

Osmosis is the flow of water across a semipermeable membrane from a low salt concentration (dilute) towards a higher salt concen-tration until a balance is reached on both sides. Water is attracted

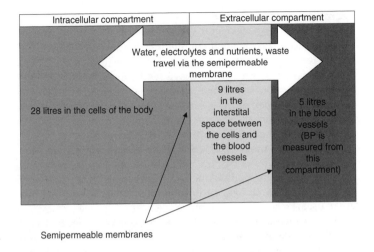

Intracellular compartment	Extracellular compartment

Water, electrolytes and nutrients, waste travel via the semipermeable membrane

28 litres in the cells of the body

9 litres in the interstital space between the cells and the blood vessels

5 litres in the blood vessels (BP is measured from this compartment)

Semipermeable membranes

Fig. 6.2 Diagram of how fluid is divided in the body, based on a 70-kg man.

to the higher concentration of salt because the higher salt level acts as a magnet to draw water through the holes in the semipermeable membrane (Davies 2010; Jenkins et al., 2010). Diffusion is the flow of salts (dissolved in water) from a higher concentration area towards a lower concentration until it is equally spread on both sides of the semipermeable membrane. In diffusion, the substance will travel down the concentration gradient.

As human beings are essentially walking, giant 42-l bags of fluid, it is important that this fluid is topped up and maintained through eating and drinking. To maintain hydration, it is essential to drink fluid to replace what is lost from metabolism and the waste products that are produced. If there is inadequate intake of fluids, then a person can become dehydrated and become unwell. Dehydration is one of the causes of *hypovolaemic shock*, which may lead to AKI (CCSI, 2009; NCEPOD, 2009). It has been found that at least 50% of AKI cases in hospital could have been prevented. If AKI does occur in a patient, the correct treatment can reverse the effects, and Perkins and Kisiel (2005) suggest that 94% of AKI survivors can return to a normal life without having to depend on dialysis.

Excretion of waste via the kidneys

Within the kidneys are millions of nephrons surrounded and entwined with a vast blood supply, which allows the kidneys to reabsorb water and salts or excrete waste in the form of urea. Urea is a nitrogenous waste broken down by the liver. It is toxic to the body and therefore sent to the kidneys for excretion in the form of urine. This complex process is called autoregulation. Once urea is produced, it travels via the ureters to the bladder where it will be passed out when a person performs micturition.

If the body is unable to excrete urine because the kidneys are failing to work properly, urea will build up in the body and become toxic to the body. A person can become *uremic* and may become confused, drowsy or unconscious. Other signs of uremia are nausea, hiccups or twitching.

We can measure the levels of urea by taking a specific blood sample known as urea and electrolytes (U&Es). If the urea and creatinine levels are outside normal range, it usually indicates that there is a kidney problem. NCEPOD (2009, p. 5) recommended that all emergency admissions should have their U&Es routinely checked and monitored in order to prevent 'the insidious and unrecognized onset of AKI'.

Practice point 6.2

As a nurse you may have the skills and competence to take blood samples using venepuncture, but you need to know what normal ranges are. Find out what the normal range for U&Es are.

FACTORS THAT INFLUENCE URINE OUTPUT

As discussed earlier, it is important that everyone remains well hydrated through eating and drinking. However, during acute or chronic illness, the kidney can be affected by factors that are divided into prerenal, renal (intrinsic) and postrenal causes.

Prerenal causes are problems that occur from before the kidney – for example, problems with the heart. If there is a problem with the heart (following a heart attack) and its ability to pump blood to the kidney and its blood supply, this will have

Table 6.1 Prerenal, renal and postrenal causes of renal failure.

Prerenal (before the kidney)	Renal (inside the kidney)	Postrenal (after the kidney)
Diarrhoea Vomiting Not drinking/eating	Many types of drugs Tumours in the kidney Pylonephritis	Obstruction – tumours Blockages from clots or pus Clamped or kinked urinary catheters
Fasting (nil orally) Heart (pump) problems Sepsis Liver problems Burns Haemorrhage	Abscess Thrombosis Stenosis	Enlarged prostate

a knock on effect on the kidneys, which will not be receiving enough oxygen and blood to keep working. The kidneys, starved of oxygen and a good blood supply, start to fail and will show signs of AKI (Table 6.1).

Renal causes often occur from damage directly inside the kidney. This can be from swellings or tumours that block the kidneys, from urinary tract infections (UTIs) or from the many types of drugs that can be toxic to the kidney.

Postrenal causes are problems that affect the kidney from the ureters and bladder. The most common reason found in hospital is from clamped or kinked urinary catheters. An enlarged prostate in men can also block the urethra and make it painful to pass urine.

NORMAL RANGE FOR MAINTAINING HYDRATION AND URINE OUTPUT

It is recommended that adults drink/eat between 2 and 3 l of fluid per day depending on the environment that they live. For example, if you live in the Sahara Desert, where the temperatures can reach 58°C, you will need to drink more to compensate for any lost fluid from perspiration. In fact, the higher the body temperature, the more fluid will be required. For every degree above 37°C, it is estimated that an adult will require between 500 and 1000 ml of extra fluid to maintain hydration, perfusion to the kidneys and overall homeostasis.

To calculate the average urine output per hour of adults, it is necessary to know how much they weigh in kilograms (kg). In adults, adequate urine output averages 0.5–1 ml per kg per hour (0.5 ml/kg/hr). For example, a 50-kg patient weight multiplied by 0.5 ml equals 25 ml per hour; but when multiplied by 1 ml it equals 50 ml per hour. Therefore, a 50-kg patient's urine output should range between 25 and 50 ml per hour (if monitored).

An output of less than (<) 0.5 ml/kg/hr for more than 2 consecutive hours always requires intervention. This intervention may range from simply getting the patient to drink more oral fluids to providing additional hydration via an intravenous infusion. The intervention will depend on the decisions made by the registered practitioner or the medical team (CCSI, 2009).

WHAT IS A NORMAL SAMPLE OF URINE?

In normal health, urine will have a pale yellowy colour, is see-through with no debris and has no odour. When you are examining urine, look at the appearance of the sample to find out what the colour and clarity is. Be aware that certain types of foods and medications can change the colour of the urine – for example, beetroot. A cloudy sample of urine is abnormal and may indicate an infection (Marieb, 2009). A freshly voided sample of urine should not have an odour, but if left to stand will begin to produce ammonia. Infected urine classically smells of rotting fish and this smell will become more pungent if left to stand. If a patient has been starving, the urine may smell of pear drops that are associated with ketones.

HOW TO MEASURE URINE OUTPUT

As we have discussed earlier, we are made up of fluid. Fluid weighs the equivalent of 1 kg to 1000 ml (1.0 l). Therefore, we can weigh patients, soiled sheets or dressings and be able to work out how much fluid was lost (Table 6.2). We can also measure fluid by collecting fluid loss via urinary measurement bags, stoma bags or measuring in a sterile jug. When collecting any bodily fluids, it is necessary to maintain standard precautions that adhere to your local hospital or community policies (Chapter 2).

Most clinical areas have access to a weighing scale. Ensure that it is serviced and calibrated before using it to ensure accuracy. The pictures in Fig. 6.3 show a step-by-step method of measuring fluid.

Table 6.2 Converting kilograms into millilitres.

One kilogram is the equivalent of 1000 ml (or 1 l)

Kilogram	Millilitres
1.0	1000
0.9	900
0.8	800
0.7	700
0.6	600
0.5	500
0.4	400
0.3	300
0.2	200
0.1	100

Some patients will be at risk of gaining fluid too easily and will become at risk of fluid overload. Therefore, by weighing the patient every day, it is possible to find out how much extra fluid the patient is carrying around. This can be useful in renal, liver and oncology patients, as many of these patients have problems with ascites.

Recording an accurate fluid balance chart

If the registered nurse or the medical staff have asked that a fluid balance chart be maintained, it is important that the record is accurate with measurable data. Use of shorthand notations is not acceptable. It must be clearly documented as to how frequently the fluid balance data is recorded – for example, hourly, 2 hourly, 4 hourly or 12 hourly.

When using a fluid balance chart, all fluid input must be recorded. It is vital that all recordings are made using quantifiable amounts, which means that it will be necessary to know how many millilitres of fluid is in a cup of tea, for example. When recording input on the fluid balance chart, please ensure that all intake is recorded. This can include any intravenous fluids, intravenous antibiotics, nasogastric feed or medications and any oral drinks.

Recording the output is equally important. There can be output from urine, diarrhoea, vomit, nasogastric aspirate, wound dressings, stoma bags, wound drainage bags, to name but a few.

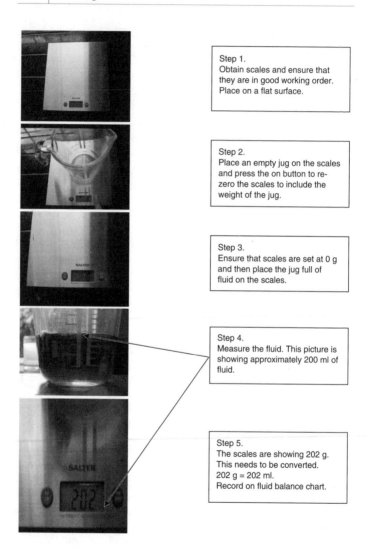

Step 1.
Obtain scales and ensure that they are in good working order. Place on a flat surface.

Step 2.
Place an empty jug on the scales and press the on button to re-zero the scales to include the weight of the jug.

Step 3.
Ensure that scales are set at 0 g and then place the jug full of fluid on the scales.

Step 4.
Measure the fluid. This picture is showing approximately 200 ml of fluid.

Step 5.
The scales are showing 202 g. This needs to be converted.
202 g = 202 ml.
Record on fluid balance chart.

Fig. 6.3 A step by step method of weighing and measuring fluids.

Some fluid balance charts include a column for a running total (also known as cumulative balance) of both the input and the output in a 24-hour period (Table 6.3a and b). Cumulative balance will indicate whether or not there are any input or output deficits over a period of days. Too much fluid intake can lead to hypervolaemia if there is renal failure and the body is unable to excrete excess fluid/wastes to keep the body in its homeostatic balance. Too little fluid can head towards hypovolaemia and this can lead to *renal failure*.

Table 6.3a 24-Hour fluid balance chart (1).

Time	Oral	IV I	IV meds	Urine	Vomit	Bowels	Stoma
08.00	Tea	Hartman's 100 ml		Toilet			
09.00		100 ml					
10.00	Coffee	100 ml	100 ml Flagyl				
11.00		85 ml					
12.00	Coffee	Tissued		Toilet		BO+	
13.00							
14.00	Tea						
15.00		Venflon sited		200 ml			
16.00			100 ml Flagyl			BO+++	
17.00	Tea						
18.00							
19.00							
20.00	Coffee			200 ml			
21.00							
22.00			100 ml Flagyl	Toilet			
23.00							
24.00							
01.00							
02.00							
03.00	Tea						
04.00				Toilet			
05.00							
06.00			100 ml Flagyl				
07.00							
Total		350 ml	400 ml	400 ml			

Table 6.3b 24-Hour fluid balance chart (2).

Time	Oral input	IV I input	IV medications	Cumulative input	Urine output	Vomit output	Bowels output	Cumulative output
08.00	Tea 100 ml	Hartman's 100 ml		200 ml	500 ml			500 ml
09.00		100 ml		300 ml				500 ml
10.00	Coffee 150 ml	100 ml	100 ml Flagyl	650 ml				500 ml
11.00		85 ml		735 ml				500 ml
12.00	Coffee 75 ml	Tissued		810 ml	200 ml		100 ml	800 ml
13.00				810 ml				800 ml
14.00	Tea 200 ml			1010 ml				800 ml
15.00		Venflon sited		1010 ml	200 ml			1000 ml
16.00	Fizzy drink 330 ml		100 ml Flagyl	1440 ml			100 ml	1100 ml
17.00	Tea 150 ml			1590 ml				1100 ml
18.00				1590 ml				1100 ml
19.00	Fizzy drink 330 ml			1920 ml	200 ml			1300 ml
20.00	Coffee 100 ml			2020 ml				1300 ml
21.00				2020 ml				1300 ml
22.00			100 ml Flagyl	2120 ml				1300 ml
23.00	Water 100 ml			2220 ml	500 ml			1800 ml
24.00				2220 ml				1800 ml
01.00				2220 ml				1800 ml
02.00				2220 ml				1800 ml
03.00	Tea 150 ml			2370 ml	200 ml			2000 ml
04.00				2370 ml				2000 ml
05.00				2370 ml				2000 ml
06.00			100 ml Flagyl	2470 ml				2000 ml
07.00	Coffee 100 ml			2570 ml				2000 ml
TOTAL	1785 ml	385 ml	400 ml	**2570 ml**	1800 mls		200 mls	**2000 mls**
Cumulative balance				**+570 ml**				

Practice point 6.3

Compare fluid balance charts (1) and (2). Look at the similarities and differences. Which chart is the more accurate fluid balance and what are the reasons for this?

Practice point 6.4

Compare the fluid balance charts that you use in your practice area to the samples within this box. What are the strengths and weaknesses of the fluid balance charts? If you find any weakness, think about ways to improve the fluid balance charts.

PERFORMING URINALYSIS USING REAGENT STRIPS

Obtaining a urine sample and performing urinalysis can be a useful aid to the medical staff in screening for potential of infection or disease (Cook, 1995).

Preparation

The following steps are involved in the preparation of the patient for sample collection.

1. Explain to the patients the reasons for testing the urine to obtain their consent and how the sample should be obtained.
2. Maintain an environment that protects their dignity and privacy.
3. Provide access to hand hygiene facilities and gloves.
4. Use sterile container to collect a midstream specimen of urine.
5. Use sterile bottle if being sent off to microbiology for a culture and sensitivity screen.
6. After collecting the sample, take a reagent strip out of its container. Ensure that the reagent strip container is in date.
7. Dip the reagent strip into the urine to cover all parts of the test strip.
8. Remove the strip by dragging the edge of the strip against the rim of the container to remove excess urine.

9. Compare the strip to the colour codes found on the container. Read each pad according to the time scale advised on the container.
10. Record results and report to the registered practitioner.

(See Table 6.4) for significance of reagent strip results.

Performing collection of catheter specimen of urine (CSU)

The following procedure must be followed while collecting catheter specimen of urine.

1. Wear gloves and protective clothing.
2. Explain to the patient the reasons for testing the urine to obtain their consent to obtain the sample.
3. Using the ANTT technique (refer to Chapter 1), open up the syringe and attach the needle.
4. Clean the catheter around the sample port using an alcohol wipe and allow it to dry.
5. Insert the needle into the sample port and pull back the syringe plunger in order to aspirate some urine.

Obtaining a midstream urine specimen

The following procedure must be followed to obtain a midstream urine specimen.

1. Explain to patient how to obtain the specimen when passing urine first time for the day.
2. Overnight urine will have accumulated in the bladder and provide the best specimen for microscopic examination.
3. The patient should start to pass urine and then stop by tensing up their pelvic floor muscles. The patient should then put the sterile receiver into the bedpan and then restart passing urine by relaxing their muscles. The sterile urine that has been collected in the sterile receiver can then be poured into a sterile specimen pot and labelled.
4. Ensure that urine sample is received at the laboratory within 2 hours of collection. If the sample is kept refrigerated at 4°C, it can be stored up to 24 hours before being examined. If the

Table 6.4 Significance of the reagent strip results.

Substance	Normal result	Abnormal result
Glucose	Negative	Positive results may signify that the blood glucose levels are high or due to reduced renal absorption. Associated with diabetes mellitus, acute pancreatitis and Cushing's syndrome
Ketones	Negative	Presence of ketones can indicate that starvation has occurred, which has resulted in the breakdown of fatty acids into the urine. Uncontrolled diabetes is another possible cause of ketones. Some drugs can cause false positives such as phenolphthalein and 1-dopa metabolites
Protein	Less than 0.5 g is normal. Trace of protein not always significant – clinical judgement	Greater than 0.5 g is viewed as clinical proteinuria. Positive protein can indicate infection, hypertension, preeclampsia or congestive cardiac failure
Blood	Negative	Four main causes of blood in urine include trauma, infection, tumours or renal stones
		False positive if menstruating. The use of stale urine and contaminated containers can give false positives
Bilirubin	Negative	Positive result may indicate liver or biliary disease. The use of stale urine can give false positives
Urobilinogen	Small amounts found in urine	A result of 33 umol/l indicates that the presence of liver abnormalities or excessive destruction of red blood cells
Nitrate	Negative	A positive result may indicate the presence of gram negative bacteria (e.g. *Escherichia Coli*). *E. Coli* is responsible for 80% of urine infections and strongly suggests the presence of a UTI

(continued)

Table 6.4 *Continued*

Substance	Normal result	Abnormal result
Leucocytes	Negative	A positive result is a useful indicator of bladder or renal infection and a full urine culture will be required to confirm this. False positives can be found where contamination from vaginal discharge and elevated glucose can decrease test results
pH	Normal range is 4.6–8.0	pH > 8.0 may indicate the presence of bacteria, usually from urea being converted to ammonia
Specific gravity – a measure of the kidney's ability to concentrate or dilute urine	Normal range 1.001–1.035	A low specific gravity may indicate hypervolaemia, renal abnormalities or diabetes insipidus
		A high specific gravity may be present in high levels of protein or dehydration

sample is left out at room temperature, then the bacteria in the urine will start to overgrow and give false result (Dougherty and Lister 2008).

URINE OUTPUT: APPLYING THE LOOK, LISTEN AND FEEL APPROACH

When assessing urine output, first look at the patient's urine. Look at the colour and look for any signs of debris, cloudiness, pus or blood clots. Look at the fluid balance chart (if one is being recorded) and make sure that it is an accurate record of oral intake, intravenous intake (input) and what has been excreted from urinary catheters, defaecation, vomit, drains or stomas (output). Listen to the patients and find out from them when they last went to the toilet and whether or not they experience pain or stinging when they urinate. This may be an early sign of a urinary infection. If assisting a patient with a bed bath, take time to feel the skin and check whether it is warm, cold or oedematous. Patients may complain of pain in their lower abdomen because of a full bladder and may be have urinary retention. This should prompt further investigation so that the patients can be treated as quickly as possible.

Practice point 6.5a

Mr Walker is a 55-year-old gentleman who was admitted to the medical assessment unit last night. He has been suffering from severe diarrhoea and vomiting and is being treated for gastroenteritis. The doctor inserted an IVI and a urinary catheter. The doctor has requested that a 24-hour fluid balance be recorded. Mr Walker weighs 70 kg. Calculate how much urine Mr Walker should drain via his catheter every hour.

Practice point 6.5b

It is now several hours since Mr Walker was admitted. You are asked to record his vital signs. On doing so you notice that his BP has dropped from 120/70 to 100/60. His heart rate has increased from 90 bpm to 120 bpm. His respiration rate has increased from 15 to 20. His temperature is normal. His urine output via his catheter for the previous 2 hours has been 15 and 25 ml.

What action should you take in the first instance? What could his potential problems be? How can you assist the nurse and the doctor?

CONCLUSION

In this chapter, we have briefly discussed the anatomy and physiology of the kidneys in the context of urine output regulation. Measuring and documenting urine output may be a useful clinical observation when caring for patients who are acutely unwell and provide vital warning signs of a failing kidney. Urine output and fluid balance measurements are an essential element of the patient's vital signs. A basic knowledge of how the kidney is regulated and the factors that influence renal function aids in performing a fluid balance assessment competently. Early U&E sampling will alert the nurse to early signs of AKI and will also ensure that patients are treated in a timely manner.

Observing and recording of urine output, urine colour and odour using the look, listen and feel approach will provide a comprehensive assessment. It is essential to inform and gain consent from the patient prior to performing urinary catheter care and it is also necessary to follow infection prevention procedures and document accurate recordings.

REFERENCES

Adam SK and Osborne S (2001). *Critical Care Nursing: Science and Practice*. Oxford, Oxford Medical Publications.

Cook R (1995). Urinalysis. *Nursing Standard* **9**(28), 32–37.

Critical Care Skills Institute (CCSI) (2009). *Acute Illness Management. AIM Course Manual*. Greater Manchester, Critical Care Skills Institute. www.gmcriticalcareskillsinstitute.org.uk.

Davies A (2009). How to manage patients with acute kidney injury. *Journal of Renal Nursing* **1**(3), 119–122.

Davies A (2010). How to perform fluid assessments in patients with renal disease. *Journal of Renal Nursing* **2**(2), 76–79.

Dougherty L and Lister S (2008). *The Royal Marsden Hospital Manual of Clinical Nursing Procedures*. 7th edn. Oxford, Wiley-Blackwell.

Fillingham S and Douglas S (2004). *Urological Nursing*. 3rd edn. London, Bailliere Tindall.

Jenkins G, Kemnitz C, and Tortora G (2010). *Anatomy and Physiology. From Science to Life*. 2nd edn. Asia, John Wiley and Sons.

Marieb EN (2009). *Essentials of Human Anatomy & Physiology*. 9th edn. San Francisco, Pearson Benjamin Cummings.

National Confidential Enquiry into Patient Outcome and Death (NCEPOD) (2009). *Acute Kidney Injury: Adding Insult to Injury*. London. NCEPOD www.ncepod.org.uk.

O'Callaghan C and Brenner B (2001). *The Kidney at a Glance*. Blackwell Publishing Ltd. Oxford.

Perkins C and Kisiel (2005). Utilising physiological knowledge to care for acute renal failure. *British Journal of Nursing* **14**(14), 768–773.

Tortora G and Derrickson B (2006). *Principles of Anatomy and Physiology*. 11th edn. United states of America. John Wiley and Sons.

Waugh A and Grant A (2001). *Ross and Wilson Anatomy and Physiology in Health and Illness*. 9th edn. London, Churchill Livingstone.

Pain: The Fifth Vital Sign

7

INTRODUCTION

Pain has been acknowledged as the fifth vital sign by the Royal Colleges of Surgeons and Anaesthetists (1996) and therefore it should form an integral component in performing and monitoring a patient's vital signs. Underpinning knowledge of the anatomy and physiology of the central nervous system is essential in monitoring the vital signs of patients who are in pain and therefore pain assessment is a fundamental part of recording and monitoring the patients' vital signs.

LEARNING OUTCOMES

By the end of this chapter, you will be able to discuss the following:

❑ The anatomy and physiology of pain transmission
❑ Definitions of acute and chronic pain
❑ The physiological consequences of pain
❑ The assessment and management of pain
❑ World Health Organisation pain ladder
❑ Pharmacological pain management strategies

THE ANATOMY AND PHYSIOLOGY OF PAIN TRANSMISSION

Wood (2008) described acute pain as being a physiological response that warns us of a threat or danger to the body. This physiological response comes from the nervous system that directs and manages the functions of all the cells and tissues within the body.

Vital Signs for Nurses: An Introduction to Clinical Observations, First Edition.
Joyce Smith and Rachel Roberts.
© 2011 Joyce Smith and Rachel Roberts. Published 2011 by Blackwell Publishing Ltd.

The nervous system is made up of three main divisions: the central nervous system, the peripheral nervous system and the autonomic nervous system (Frizzell, 2001).

The delicate structures of the central nervous system require a defence mechanism that comes from the bony structures of the skull and the vertebral column. The skull protects the brain, and the vertebral column protects the spinal cord. Three protective membranes known as the *meninges* encircle the spinal cord and the brain (Fig. 7.1). The inner layer is known as the *Pia mater*, which is made up of clear, transparent connective tissue that adheres to the surface of the spinal cord and brain. The middle layer is called the *Arachnoid mater* because it gives the impression of being like a spider's web. The outer layer is known as the *Dura mater* because

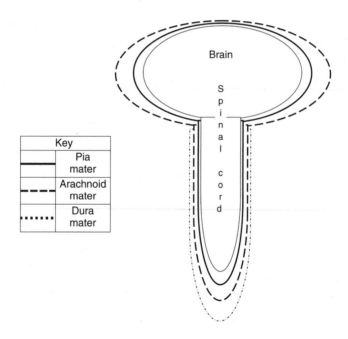

Fig. 7.1 Hand-drawn picture of the brain and spinal cord with meninges by Rachel Roberts. Reproduced by Helen Smith.

it is made up of tough connective tissue. The meninges 'PAD' the central nervous system (Tortora and Nielsen, 2009).

The space between the wall of the vertebral channel and the dura mater is the *epidural space*, and anaesthetists are trained to administer epidural analgesia into this space using a fine bore indwelling catheter via a Tuohy needle to provide pain relief. Nurses may be asked to monitor and record the vital signs of patients who are using epidural analgesia. Between the dura mater and the arachnoid mater is the *subdural space* and between the arachnoid mater and the pia mater is the *subarachnoid space*. The subarachnoid space also contains cerebrospinal fluid that provides nutrients and also acts as a shock absorber for the brain and spinal cord (Tortora and Nielsen, 2009). Nurses may be asked to monitor and record the vital signs of patients with symptoms of photophobia or headache. These signs may indicate a subarachnoid haemorrhage and will require urgent medical intervention.

The central nervous system is made up of the brain and the spinal cord. The spinal cord is the conduit that links the peripheral nervous system to the central nervous system via the essential units of the nervous system known as *neurons*. Neurons (or nerve cells) relay information and activity through sensory and motor responses (Fig. 7.2). It is estimated that there are over 100 billion interconnecting neurons within the nervous system (Knight and Nigam, 2008). Each neuron is made up of a cell body, axons and dendrites. Electrical and chemical impulses travel along each neuron relaying messages to and from the central and peripheral nervous systems. Axons always carry the electrical or chemical impulse away from the cell body and the dendrites conduct the impulse towards the cell body (Morton et al., 2005). When the impulse travels to the end of the axon, the message is relayed to the next neuron through the release of neurotransmitters that diffuse across the synapse. There are different sizes of neurons, and some are myelinated and others are not. Myelin is a lipid-protein sheath that acts as an insulator to keep the impulse from dispersing away, and nerves covered with myelin have an increase in the speed of the impulse (Huether and McCance, 2000).

The areas of the central nervous system that control and interpret painful stimuli include the limbic system, reticular formation,

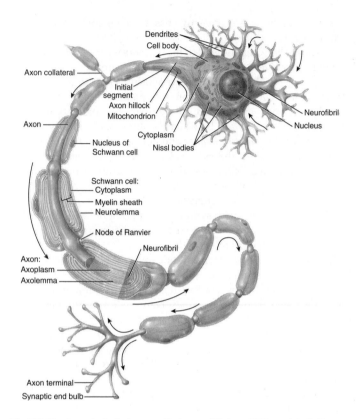

Fig. 7.2 Structure of a typical neuron. Tortora and Nielsen, 2009; reprinted with permission from John Wiley and Sons Inc.

thalamus, hypothalamus, medulla and cortex. The medulla and the hypothalamus activate the 'flight or fight' responses and release corticosteroids and affect the cardiovascular response (Huether and McCance, 2000).

There are special neurons that have been designed to detect painful stimuli within the body, which are called *nociceptors*. Noxious or harmful stimuli may originate from mechanical, thermal or chemical causes. Mechanical stimuli may be triggered by inflammation, swelling, surgical incision or growth of tumours that leads to pressure on tissues and structures within the body. Thermal stimuli may be triggered by a burn or scald to the skin, such as sunburn or handling a hot pan. Chemical nociceptors may be activated from the release of excitatory neurotransmitters, such as substance P when tissue ischaemia or infection is present. It is a neuropeptide that transmits pain and can be found in the spinal cord, brain and gastrointestinal tract. Other noxious chemicals that stimulate pain include prostaglandin, serotonin and histamine to name but a few (Huether and McCance, 2000; Wood, 2008).

When the nociceptors of C fibre and A-delta fibres are stimulated or exposed to a noxious or harmful stimulus (such as a scald from boiling water on the skin), they fire an impulse that travels along the neuron from the peripheral nerves to the central nervous system via the dorsal horn of the spinal cord (Fig. 7.3). From the spinal cord, the message may travel to the brain where the painful stimuli are processed and perception of pain is recognised (Wood, 2008). Being able to perceive pain acts as a warning sign to cell and tissue

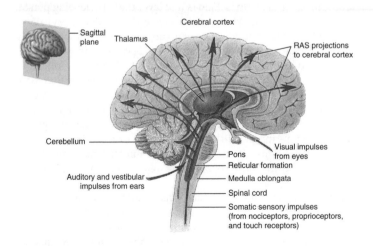

Fig. 7.3 Anatomy of the spinal cord and the spinal nerves. Tortora and Nielsen, 2008; reprinted with permission from John Wiley and Sons Inc.

damage and this is called *Nociception*. McCaffery and Pasero (1999) outline four basic processes involved in nociception and these are transduction, transmission, perception and modulation.

Perception of pain depends on how the brain interprets the information from the pain impulse. The brain modulates or adapts the noxious stimuli so that we can perceive pain to be either acute or chronic. The brain can adjust the noxious stimuli by releasing inhibitory neuropeptides such as endorphin and encephalin (naturally occurring opiates) along the neuron to reduce the perception of pain (Huether and McCance, 2000).

DEFINITIONS OF PAIN

It is not surprising that the International Association for the Study of Pain (IASP, 2007) has defined pain on its website (www.iasp-pain.org) as 'An unpleasant sensory and emotional experience with actual or potential tissue damage, or described in terms of such damage'. The IASP group emphasises that pain is always subjective or personal to an individual and this makes it complex for nurses to assess and manage effectively. Within nursing circles, an influential quote for defining pain is 'Pain is whatever the experiencing person says it is, and exists whenever he says it does' (McCaffery, 1999). This infers that pain is a unique experience that cannot be fully comprehended by another human being. Because pain is a difficult concept to define with many aspects to it, the Royal College of Surgeons and Royal College of Anaesthetists (1996) state that 'pain is a subjective experience that can be perceived directly only by the sufferer. It is a multi-dimensional phenomenon that can be described by pain, location, intensity, temporal aspects, quality impact and meaning. Pain does not occur in isolation but in specific human being in psychosocial, economic and cultural contexts that influence the meaning, experience and verbal and non verbal expression of pain'.

Pain is divided into two main classifications – acute or chronic (Dougherty and Lister, 2008). Acute pain has been described as being triggered by an event, with sudden onset, and as painful areas well defined that can be relieved with treatment. Acute pain may be triggered by an event (for example, breaking your leg after slipping on ice or snow). Acute pain has a sudden onset, but the painful areas will be well defined and may be relieved with analgesic treatment. There is also a psychological aspect to pain because many patients will experience increased levels of anxiety whilst in pain. If treated promptly, acute pain is associated with full recovery, although the time frame from onset to recovery may last up to six months. Chronic pain has been defined as a persistent pain having lasted at least 6 months and can last months or even years. Chronic pain can have an insidious onset and the pain may be continuous or intermittent and usually increases over time. Complete relief from chronic pain is not usually possible, and psychologically this is associated with a sense of helplessness and hopelessness that may result in the development of depression (Huether and McCance, 2000).

Practice point 7.1

In the table below write down four acute and chronic conditions that you may have experienced or seen in health care.

Acute pain conditions	Chronic pain conditions

In recent times, it has been acknowledged that acute and chronic pain are not two distinct entities but may signify a continuum of combined pain mechanisms that vary in duration (Macintyre et al., 2010). Kehlet et al. (2006) studied cases of persisting pain post-surgery and suggested that this can develop into post-surgical chronic pain as a result of either ongoing inflammation or as a symptom of neuropathic pain from surgical injury to major peripheral nerves. Pain is common in older people because of the chronic medical and skeletal problems such as diabetes, angina, chronic obstructive pulmonary disease, fractures, rheumatoid arthritis and osteoarthritis. However, pain should not be accepted as an inevitable consequence of ageing, and healthcare staff in nursing and residential care homes should observe for signs of pain in their residents and seek to support them with treatment (Swann, 2010). The Royal College of Physicians (2007, p. 2) stated that 'pain is under-recognised and under-treated in older people'. The assessment of pain becomes challenging for the nurse or doctor when the older person presents with severe cognitive impairment, communication difficulties or language or cultural barriers.

It has been recognised that pain can lead to increased levels of anxiety that in turn can affect sleep and rest patterns. Pain may affect levels of appetite and within health care can lead to delays in recovery, with increased complications and a rise in healthcare costs. Nurses play a pivotal role in the assessment and management of a patient's acute pain. It is essential for nursing staff to address acute pain, as there is the potential for acute pain to progress into chronic pain (Carr and Goudas, 1999).

PAIN ASSESSMENT STRATEGIES

Pain is a multidimensional process that includes the physiological, psychological and social factors that may affect the patient's perception of pain. The communication and observational skills of the nurses cannot be underestimated in their assessment of a patient who has acute pain. Knowledge and understanding of the most appropriate pain assessment tool including the physiological and psychological factors will ultimately inform the patient's pain assessment and management plan. As succinctly described by Swann (2010), pain is subjective and unique to each individual. Although nursing staff are often the first person to assess a patient's pain, Haigh (2001) focused on the assessment of pain by multidisciplinary team members during their initial contact with the patient. Interestingly, the study revealed that only 64% of nurses stated that they would assess a patient's pain prior to commencing care or treatment compared to 80% of physiotherapists and 88% of doctors who routinely assessed the patient's pain. The poor response by nurses to pain assessment prior to commencing care or treatment is in line with the findings by Manias et al. (2002), who identified that during 12 periods of observation, nurses did not assess the patient's pain before their planned care or treatment. The findings from the study by Haigh (2001) suggest that although pain assessment was clearly identified as important, each discipline was recording their assessment of pain in their own records, therefore a lack of effective communication and the potential for inconsistencies of pain management. MacLellan (2006) advocates a multidisciplinary team approach that involves each discipline taking responsibility for assessing and documenting the patient's pain. Pain assessment tools are only one dimensional in assessing the patient's experience of acute pain; the physiological response to pain also informs the assessment process.

The patients' self-report of their pain experience is the most reliable indicator of their pain because they describe the location, intensity and duration of their pain. The gold standard is to always ask the patients about their pain; however, previous studies have highlighted a reluctance by patients to report their pain because they perceive staff to have competing demands on their time and appear to be very busy (Manias et al., 2002). Accurate pain assessment has been identified by Kozier et al (2008) as central to effective pain management; Cousins and Carr (2010) state that it is a fundamental human right. Beretta (2008) reiterates that assessment is an ongoing process that gathers information that is objective and subjective. An accurate assessment of acute pain is crucial to providing an individualised plan of care based on the patient's pain experience. It is recommended that a pain assessment be carried out at the same time as other routine vital signs monitoring. Pain should be assessed using a recognised pain assessment tool 'at rest' and then 'on movement' to compare the difference (Dougherty and Lister, 2008). The purpose of pain assessment tools is to translate the subjective experience of pain into objective numbers or descriptors.

Many patients in acute pain (e.g. on admission to accident and emergency or postoperatively) are able to articulate their needs, and therefore a verbal or numerical assessment tool will provide sufficient information for the patient's initial assessment. Verbal Rating Scales (VRS) comprise of four to five words that describe pain and the patients choose a word that best describes their pain. Visual analogue scales (VAS) consist of a straight line and the

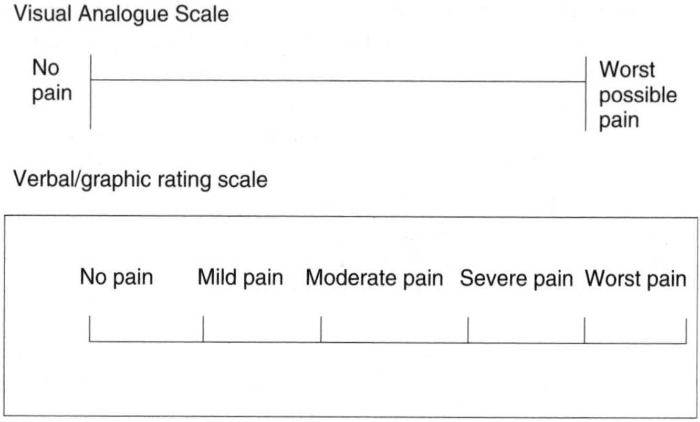

Visual Analogue Scale

No pain		Worst possible pain

Verbal/graphic rating scale

No pain	Mild pain	Moderate pain	Severe pain	Worst pain

Fig. 7.4 Samples of verbal and numerical pain assessment scales.

number corresponding to the patient's mark on the line is the pain intensity score. Numeric rating scale (NRS) consists of a numerical scale 0–10 in which no pain is scored at 0, and 10 is intense severe pain; whichever number the patient chooses is the intensity score (see Fig. 7.4).

Single dimensional scales can be utilised quickly and are often incorporated as part of the chart that records the patient's vital signs.

Example of a Verbal Rating Scale 0–3

Rating of pain	Score
None	0
Mild	1
Moderate	2
Severe	3

The advantage of using a unidimensional tool is that it is a quick and simple tool that is normally used in assessing acute pain and the patient decides the intensity of pain. The disadvantages are that it is not always a reliable tool when assessing the pain experience of patients with severe learning disabilities or cognitive impairment, because they are often unable to articulate the intensity of their pain (Davies and Evans, 2001; Kingston and Bailey, 2009).

Pain is consistently underdiagnosed or -treated in patients who have a learning disability or severe cognitive impairment (Abbey et al., 2004; McAuliffe et al., 2008). Assessment tools that rely on the patients being able to verbalise their pain have been highlighted by Davies and Evans (2001) as ineffective tools for patients who have severe learning disabilities. A review of pain assessment tools by Kingston and Bailey (2009) and their colleagues from the community learning disability team identified that a protocol was required to provide healthcare staff with a tool that would recognise the pain of people with a learning disability. A review of all pain assessment tools including multidimensional tools found that they were unsuitable and needed to be adapted to address the assessment of people with a learning disability. The authors developed a chronic and acute pain assessment tool that included a pain story (to help individuals to talk about their pain), a pain diary and a body map. The protocol was reviewed by service users with varying degrees of disabilities and communication skills. Following feedback from service users and a period of consultation, the acute pain assessment tool and the pain story were integrated to reduce duplication. The assessment tool has been disseminated throughout the community to other service providers including the acute and primary care trust.

A literature review by McAuliffe et al. (2008) identified barriers to successful pain assessment in older adults with dementia. The barriers identified included a lack of recognition, insufficient education and pain assessment tools not being routinely used. The authors highlight that a reluctance to use pain assessment tools may be because the existing tools are deficient in assessing the patient's pain. A literature review by While and Jocelyn (2009) focused on observational pain scales that could be utilised by district nurses assessing patients with dementia. The authors examined four observational tools with the aim of assessing their validity in a community nursing environment. The authors advocate the Non-communicative Patients Pain Assessment Instrument (NOPPAIN) as the assessment tool required minimal training and provided a valid measurement tool for people who are unable to communicate their pain experience. It appears from previous studies that pain assessment is a complex process and the various tools that are available do not always address the individualised needs of patients who are experiencing acute pain.

THE PHYSIOLOGICAL CONSEQUENCES OF ACUTE PAIN

Acute pain is a stimulus that triggers a physiological response by the body to cope with the effect of the stimulus (Walker et al., 2004). Tortora and Derrickson (2009) describe a stimulus as potentially causing a reaction that results in a stressor on the body. A stressor arises from an individual's assessment of a mismatch between the demands made upon them and their ability to cope. Cannon (1932) described that the reaction to a potential threat resulted in a 'fight or flight' response. The model of physiological and behavioural response to stress was developed by Hans Selye (1956), who included the concept of the fight and flight reaction into his physiological model of stress. Selye called his model the general adaptation syndrome (GAS) in which three stages are identified in the body's response to stress. The first stage is the alarm stage (shock) and the body activates a 'fight or flight' response reacting to what it perceives as a potential threat. The second stage is resistance when hormones within the body are released to maintain the resistance to stress and finally the third stage is when the body is depleted of its resources, resulting in a state of exhaustion (Walker et al., 2004; Tortora and Derrickson, 2009).

In response to stress, the body's homeostasis mechanism is affected, which in turn results in physiological changes. As the sympathetic nervous system releases adrenalin, blood is inhibited for non-essential systems – for example, the digestive and urinary systems, also including the skin – as this will provide more blood flow to the brain and muscles. Adrenaline will increase the heart rate, and as the heart is stressed, it increases the cardiac output to meet the demands of the body. The blood pressure will also be raised as blood flow to the left ventricle takes place in diastole – increasing the heart rate decreases diastole filling time and there is an increased need for oxygen because the myocardium (muscle of the heart) is working harder. For patients who have existing cardiac problems, the stress on the heart may potentially create further problems (Marieb, 2009). A reduction in blood flow to the kidneys triggers the release of renin–angiotensin and aldosterone that causes the kidneys to retain sodium and results in water retention, thereby increasing the blood pressure. At the same time that adrenaline is released, the liver converts glucagon to glucose to prepare the body for the perceived threat. The respiratory rate increases as the bronchioles dilate to allow more air and oxygen into the lungs (Marieb, 2009; Tortora and Derrickson, 2009). Cortisol, a hormone that aids the metabolic rate, is also released into the bloodstream.

The patient's vital signs will respond to the physiological changes caused by acute pain. The patient may have a raised heart rate and an increased oxygen demand. The respiratory rate will be raised and people in pain may take shallow breaths and have ineffective coughing that will lead to sputum retention. A reduced amount of oxygen because of the increased respiratory rate and consequently decreased lung volumes will result in the patient becoming hypoxic. As blood is diverted from the skin, the patient may have cool peripheries that are slightly cyanosed. The smooth muscle is affected and hence gastric emptying and reduced motility may result in the patient complaining of nausea or vomiting. Lack of adequate nutrition will lead to poor wound healing and reduced mobility, increasing the risk of deep vein thrombosis. Blood sugar levels are raised because cortisol (hydrocortisone) affects carbohydrate and protein metabolism (Marieb, 2009). Cortisol also decreases the immune function and can delay wound healing (postoperative pain). It is also possible that an increased bladder sphincter tone may lead to urinary retention and fluid and electrolyte changes, affecting the urine output as a result of increased sodium and water reabsorption (Park et al., 2000). Ultimately, unrelieved pain leads to fatigue, nausea and loss of appetite, and the patient may become depressed, and acute pain may progress to chronic pain if it is not addressed.

Practice point 7.2

A patient is admitted to your practice area with acute appendicitis. Using your local physiological observation chart, record the following observations:

BP 150/80, HR 130, RR 28, SpO_2 91%, Temperature 38.

The patient is complaining of severe pain and feels nauseous. What *other factors* will you observe to inform the pain assessment? What action will you take to manage the patient and what type of pain relief would you consider?

WORLD HEALTH ORGANISATION (WHO) PAIN LADDER

The WHO (1996) has developed a three-stepped ladder for cancer pain relief, although this stepped approach has also been adopted in acute settings. To achieve pain relief, analgesics should be administered regularly (by the clock) and not on an adhoc basis. This prevents huge peaks and troughs in pain relief and the overall use of pharmokinetics is more effective. After assessing a patient's pain score, the right level of analgesia must be administered. Too little will not provide relief but increase the patient's pain and anxiety and too much could lead to potential fatal side effects. Figure 7.5 shows an adapted WHO pain ladder.

The three-stepped analgesia ladder is simple to use against a 0–3 numerical pain score. While completing vital signs of respiration, pulse, blood pressure and temperature, the nurse can ask the patient 'Are you in any pain?' The awake patient will answer 'Yes' or 'No' to this initial question. If the patient confirms pain, the nurse can then ask 'Is your pain mild, moderate or severe?' If the reply is 'Severe', then the nurse can look at other behavioural and nonverbal cues and discuss the location and quality of the pain. The nurse can then record on the physiological chart the pain score of 3 and review the prescribed analgesic options. Remember to compare the pain score at rest and at movement as previously discussed.

However, it must be noted that Jadad and Browman (1995) performed a systematic review of studies (1982–1995) to evaluate the effectiveness of the WHO pain ladder and concluded that there

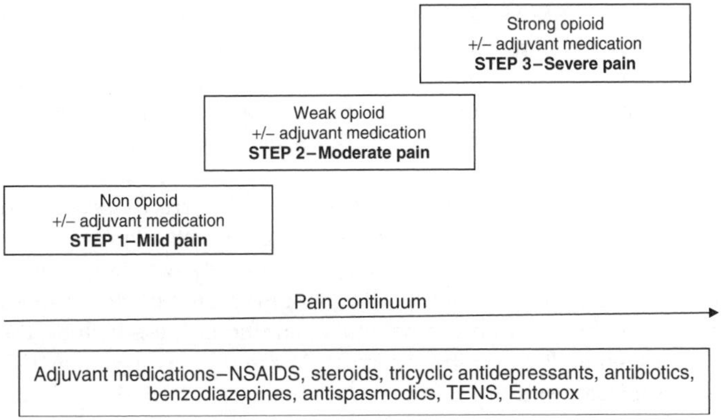

Fig. 7.5 World Health Organisation pain ladder. Adapted by Rachel Roberts and Jill Din.

was insufficient evidence to prove its effectiveness until carefully controlled trials were done. More recently, Ferreira et al. (2006) performed another systematic review (1982–2004) and came to the same conclusion. Despite the limited evidence supporting the effectiveness of the WHO pain ladder, it remains a popular system for management of pain within the clinical setting.

Practice point 7.3

From the list of drugs below, identify whether these would be mild, moderate or severe analgesics or adjuvant medications in line with the WHO analgesic ladder.

Alfentanil, amitriptiline, aspirin, bupivocaine, carbomazipine, codeine, dexamethsone, diamorphine, diazepam, fentanyl, gabapentin, GTNspray, hydrocortisone, ibrufen, ketorolac, lignocaine, methadone, morphine, MST, oromorph, oxycodone, paracetamol, pethidine, prednisolone, remifentanil and tramadol.

PHARMACOLOGICAL PAIN MANAGEMENT STRATEGIES

Analgesics are medicines that relieve pain and are divided into two main groups: opioids and non-opioids (The British Medical

Association (BMA), 2005). Opioids are generally suitable for moderate-to-severe pain and non-opioid drugs are suitable for muscular–skeletal pain-related conditions. Analgesics have been found to be more effective in preventing pain when administered regularly and by the clock (British National Formulary (BNF), 2009).

The registered nurse must only administer correctly prescribed medication, and guidance on prescribing correctly can be found on the British National Formulary website, www.bnf.org. There are various routes through which analgesics can be administered and are dependant on the patient's condition. These include the oral, parenteral, rectal, transdermal, intramuscular injection (IM) and continuous infusion, intravenous bolus or, alternatively, intravenous infusion. Care must be taken to prescribe appropriately for the elderly. Age does affect renal clearance and therefore many ageing patients can become at risk of renal failure due to nephrotoxic medications (BNF, 2009). Further information regarding prescribing for the elderly can be found in the national service framework for older people (Department of Health (DH), 2001).

Morphine is recognised as the gold standard of opioid therapy and can be administered via multiple routes of administration. However, opioids have many unpleasant side effects such as respiratory depression, cough suppression, nausea and vomiting, constipation and urinary retention. The side effects may be managed by administering the correct dose and monitoring the respiration rate and by providing anti-emetics and laxatives (McMahon and Koltzenburg, 2006). Although vital signs monitoring is essential for monitoring any analgesic effect, particular vigilance is required with patients who receive analgesia directly to the central nervous system via the epidural route, the intravenous route using patient-controlled analgesia (PCA) devices or as intravenous bolus.

EPIDURAL ANALGESIA

Administration of analgesia into the epidural space via an indwelling catheter is known as *epidural analgesia* (ANZCA and the Faculty of Medicine, 2005; Dougherty and Lister, 2008). The indwelling catheter is normally inserted by a competent practitioner (usually an anaesthetist) via the lumbar or the thoracic route. The epidural space is found between the dura mater and the walls of the vertebral canal. The epidural space extends from the base of the skull to the sacrum. The epidural space is identified by feeling for bony landmarks on the spine and pelvis. A Tuohy needle and syringe containing a small volume of local anaesthetic is injected into the skin and the interspinous ligament. It is advanced slowly, until resistance is no longer felt, indicating that the tip of the needle is in the epidural space. A fine catheter is then threaded through the needle into the epidural space and the needle is removed. In January 2008, the National Institute for Health and Clinical Excellence (NICE, 2008) issued guidance regarding the role of ultrasound in the insertion of epidurals and suggested that it aids in increasing safety on insertion.

The area of analgesic effect is dependant on the site of insertion in relation to surgery (Weetman and Allison, 2006), and Table 7.1 outlines the possible locations for the surgical sites.

Epidurals may be used for acute or palliative analgesic purposes (Day, 2001). There is a plethora of literature relating to epidural analgesia used in post-operative maternity and surgical patients (Bird and Wallis, 2002); Cox (2007) endorsed thoracic epidural analgesia as a safe and effective way to manage pain in patients who have undergone major thoracic surgery. However, there are some contraindications for epidurals that the nurse must be aware of. Epidurals should only be administered to a patient who gives consent and fully understands the procedure (DH, 2001; Nursing and Midwifery Council (NMC), 2006). Other contraindications include septicaemia due to the increased risk of spreading the infection into the spinal system; leading to

Table 7.1 Epidural locations for surgical sites.

Epidural locations for surgical sites
T6–T9 thoracic surgery
T7–T10 upper abdominal surgery
T9–L1 lower abdominal surgery
L1–L4 hip and knee surgery

Adapted from Dougherty and Lister, 2008.

increased risks of epidural abscess, meningitis or neurological damage; deformed spine or gross obesity that makes it difficult to site the catheter; neurological disease; coagulopathies and patients at higher risk of spinal catheter infections as in insulin-dependent diabetics or the immunocompromised (Day, 2001; Weetman and Allison, 2006). Epidurals should only be used in areas where the nursing and medical staff have been trained and assessed as competent to use them in areas such as theatres, critical care, maternity, surgical wards or in palliative care. The benefits of epidural analgesia include enhanced pain relief and reduced postoperative complications such as chest infections, nausea and vomiting, deep vein thrombosis, constipation and delayed bowel movements. It has been suggested that epidural analgesia also reduces the stress response that improves recovery and survival rates and decreases hospital stay (Keht, 1997; Weetman and Allison, 2006).

Patients with epidural analgesia require vital signs monitoring immediately post-insertion and throughout its use. Different trusts have their own guidance and policies regarding epidural observations; so please refer to your own organisational policies. Dougherty and Lister (2008) recommend that vitals signs are to be recorded immediately post-insertion to monitor for signs of hypotension (due to vasodilatation of the vessels) or respiratory depression (due to opioid analgesia). On return to the ward area, observations should be completed hourly for at least 4 hours, and if the patient remains stable, then this can be reduced to 4 hourly for 24 hours. Motor block should be measured by assessing the patient's ability to move the lower limbs including legs, knees and feet using the nationally recognised Bromage Scale. This measures the degree of block and is useful in the early detection of an epidural haematoma. A grade 1 block is when the patient has free movement of legs and feet; a grade 2 block is when there is a partial block and the patient is able to flex the knees with free movement of feet; a grade 3 block is almost complete block and the patient is unable to flex the knees but has free movement of the feet and a grade 4 block is a complete block when the patient is unable to move the legs or feet. Sedation scoring should also be completed when performing a pain assessment in case the analgesia is causing respiratory depression. The epidural site should be observed for any signs of infection and inflammation using a visual infusion phlebitis (VIP) score and the values recorded. Monitor the patient for any signs of dural puncture, which include headache, nausea and vomiting. Any concerns about the epidural site or infusion should be discussed with either the Acute Pain team or the anaesthetist who inserted the epidural catheter.

PCA is widely used internationally for the treatment of acute post-operative pain. PCA allows the patients to administer to themselves a small, fixed, prescribed dose by pressing a button attached to the PCA infusion pump and timing device (Dougherty and Lister, 2008; Lindley et al., 2009). Patient education and ongoing support are necessary to ensure that the device is used correctly by the patient. PCA should only be used in patients who consent to its use, with no neurological or dexterity problems.

However, in recent times, there have been studies that challenge the role of PCA. Lindley et al. (2009) compared the effectiveness of fentanyl iontophoretic transdermal system with the PCA, and nurses found the iontophoretic system simpler and easier to use. The transdermal iontophoresis is still patient controlled but uses a transdermal patch that is similar in size to a credit card. It contains approximately 80 doses of fentanyl and the patch is placed on the patient's outer arm or chest. The patient activates a button that will deliver 40 µg of fentanyl with a 10-minute lock out. The patch will operate for 24 hours or until all the doses have been used, whichever comes first (Layzell, 2008). Comparison of PCA and intramuscular injections (IM) did not demonstrate any significant differences between them, although patients with PCA took 4.5 hours longer to mobilise than those with IM analgesia (Snell et al., 1997).

LOOK, LISTEN AND FEEL

It is important to support a pain assessment by observing for nonverbal clues using the look, listen and feel approach because patients have the potential to be in pain but may not always articulate to healthcare professionals that they are in pain.

Look at the patient's facial expressions because grimacing, sighing, and crying or even anger may be signs of discomfort and pain. Look at the patient's skin, as they may begin to pale and peripherally shut down if they are experiencing severe pain. Observe the posture of the patient. Sometimes patients pace up and down because this distracts them from their pain or others will avoid movement because this increases their pain. Some patients hold on to the area that hurts to protect it, being reluctant to reposition or mobilise. Look at any surgical or drain sites and observe for signs of infection or collections that are causing the pain.

Listen to the patients and their relatives when they tell you their concerns about pain and analgesia. Find out if some activities make the pain worse or better. As previously discussed, there is a psychological element to pain and therefore allowing patients to express their fears and anxiety about being ill or in pain and discussing or clarifying issues with them will all aid in reducing their perception of pain.

If the patient consents, *feel* the area of pain because the site may be hot and inflamed, indicating infection. Feel for any collections or abscesses. In conjunction with the pain assessment, non-verbal information about the pain experience can provide useful information to manage and treat pain more effectively.

CONCLUSION

In this chapter, we have briefly discussed the anatomy and physiology of the central nervous system in relation to pain perception. Assessing a patient's pain using a pain scoring system will aid in timely treatment and management of the pain. There are many analgesic options available to provide patients with pain relief and the WHO analgesic ladder is a useful tool to administer and titrate analgesia. When performing vital signs, a pain score should always be performed, because it is an essential element of vital signs monitoring and is the fifth vital sign.

REFERENCES

Abbey J, Piller N, De Bellis A et al. (2004). The Abbey pain scale: a 1-minute numerical indicator for people with end-stage dementia. *International Journal of Palliative Nursing*. **10**(1), 6–13.

Beretta R (2008). Assessment: the foundation of good practice. In: *Nursing Practice and Healthcare*. A Foundation Text. 5th edn. Hichcliffe S, Norman S, and Schober J (eds). London, Hodder Arnold.

Bird A and Wallis M (2002). Nursing knowledge and assessment skills in the measurement of patients receiving analgesia via epidural infusion. *Journal of Advanced Nursing* **40**(5), 522–531.

British Medical Association (BMA) (2005). *Concise Guide to Medicine and Drugs*. 2nd edn. London, Dorling Kindersley.

British National Formulary (2009). *BNF 58*. London, BMJ Group and RPS Publishing.

Cannon WB (1932). *The Wisdom of the Body*. 2nd Edn. New York, Nulton Pubs.

Carr DB and Goudas, LC (1999). Acute pain. *Lancet* **353**, 2051–2058.

Cousins MJ and Carr DB (2010). Foreword in: Macintyre PE, Schug SA, Scott DA, Visser EJ, Walker SM; APM:SE Working group of the Australian and New Zealand College pf Anaesthetists and Faculty of Pain Medicine (2010). *Acute Pain Management: Scientific Evidence*. 3rd edn. Melbourne, ANZCA & FPM.

Cox F (2007). Acute pain management after major thoracic surgery. *Nursing Times* **103**(23), 30–31.

Davies D and Evans L (2001). Assessing pain in people with profound learning disabilities. *British Journal of Nursing* **10**(8), 513–516.

Day R (2001). The use of epidural and intrathecal analgesia in palliative care. *International Journal of Palliative Nursing* **7**(8), 369–374.

Department of Health (DH) (2001). *National Service Framework for Older People*. DH.

Dougherty L and Lister S (2008). *The Royal Marsden Hospital Manual of Clinical Nursing Procedures*. 7th edn. Oxford, Wiley-Blackwell.

Ferreira K, Kimura M, and Jacobsen T (2006). The WHO analgesic ladder for cancer pain control twenty years of use: now much pain relief does one get from using it? *Supportive Care in Cancer* **14**(11), 1086–1093.

Frizzell J (2001). *Handbook of Pathophysiology*. Pennsylvania, Springhouse Cooperation.

Haigh, C (2001). Contribution of multidisciplinary team to pain management. *British Journal of Nursing* **10**(6), 370–374.

Huether SE and McCance KL (2000). *Understanding Pathophysiology*. 2nd edn. London, Mosby.

International Association for the Study of Pain (IASP) (2007). *Pain Terminology*. Accessed from www.iasp-pain.org.

Jadad A and Browman G (1995). The WHO Analgesic Ladder for cancer pain management. *Journal of American Medicine* **274**(23), 1870–1873.

Kehlet H, Jensen TS, and Woolf CJ (2006). Persistent postsurgical pain: risk factors and prevention. *Lancet* **8**(6), 514–517.

Keht (1997). *Lancet* **367**(9522), 1618–1625.

Kingston K and Bailey C (2009). Assessing the pain of people with a learning disability. *British Journal of Nursing* **18**(7), 420–423.

Knight J and Nigam Y (2008). Exploring the anatomy and physiology of aging. *Nursing Times* **104**(35), 18–19.

Kozier B, Erb G Berman A, Snyder S Lake R and Harvey S (2008). *Fundamentals of Nursing, Concepts, Process and Practice*. Essex, Pearson Education.

Layzell M (2008). Current interventions and approaches to postoperative pain management. *British Journal of Nursing* **17**(7), 414–419.

Lindley P, Pestano CR, and Gargiulo K (2009). Comparisons of postoperative pain management using two patient-controlled analgesia methods: nursing perspective. *Journal of Advanced Nursing* **65**(7), 1370–1380.

Macintyre PE, Schug SA, Scott DA, Visser EJ, Walker SM, APM: SE Working Group of the Australian and New Zealand College of Anaesthetists and Faculty of Pain Medicine (2010). *Acute Pain Management: Scientific Evidence*. 3rd edn. Melbourne, ANZCA & FPM.

MacLellan K (2006). *Management of Pain*. Cheltenham, Nelson Thornes.

Manias E, Botti, M, and Bucknall T (2002). Observation of pain assessment and management – the complexities of clinical practice. *Journal of Clinical Nursing* **11**, 724–733.

Marieb EN (2009). *Essentials of Human Anatomy and Physiology*. 9th edn. San Francisco, Pearson Benjamin Cummings.

McAuliffe L, Nay R, O'Donnell M, and Fetherstonhaugh D (2008). Pain assessment in older people with dementia: literature review. *Journal of Advanced Nursing* **65**(1), 2–10.

McCaffery M (1999). *Pain Clinical Manual*. 2nd edn. St Louis, Mosby.

McCaffery M and Pasero C (1999). *Pain Clinical Manual*. London, Mosby.

McMahon SB and Koltzenburg M (2006). *Wall and Melzack's Textbook of Pain*. 5th edn. London, Elsevier Churchill Livingstone.

Morton P, Fontaine D, Hudak C and Gallo B (2005). *Critical Care Nursing. A holistic approach*. 8th edn., Philadelphia, Lippincott, Williams and Wilkins.

National Institute for Health and Clinical Excellence (2008). *Ultrasound-guided Catheterisation of the Epidural Space*. Interventional procedure guidance 249. Issued January 2008. [Accessed June 2010]. www.nice.org.uk.

Nursing and Midwifery Council (NMC) (2006). *A-Z Advice Sheet: Consent*. [Accessed June 2010]. www.nmc/org.

Park G, Fulton B, and Senthuran S (2000). *The Management of Acute Pain*. 2nd edn. Oxford, Oxford University Press.

Royal College of Physicians (2007). *Number 8, The Assessment of Pain in Older People. National Guidelines*. [Accessed May 2010] www.rcplondon.ac.uk.

Royal College of Surgeons of England and Royal College of Anaesthetists (1996). *Commission on the Provision of Surgical Services. Report of the Working Party on Pain After Surgery*. London, Royal College of Surgeons of England.

Selye H (1956). *The Stress of Life*. New York, McGraw-Hill.

Snell CC, Fothergill-Bourbonnais F, and Durocher- Hendriks S (1997). Patients controlled analgesia and intramuscular injections: a comparison of patient pain experiences and postoperative outcomes. *Journal of Advanced Nursing* **25**, 681–690.

Swann J (2010). Pain: causes, effects and assessment. *Nursing and Residential Care* **12**(5), 212–215.

Tortora GJ and Derrickson BH (2009). *Principles of Anatomy and Physiology*, 12th edn.

Tortora and Nielsen (2009). *Principles of Human Anatomy*. 11th edn.

Walker J, Payne S, Smith, P, and Jarrett N (2004). *Psychology for Nurses and the Caring Professions*. 2nd edn. Berkshire, Open University Press. John Wiley and Sons.

Weetman C and Allison W (2006). Use of epidural analgesia in post-operative pain management. *Nursing Standard* **20**(4), 54–64.

While C and Jocelyn A (2009). Observational pain assessment scales for people with dementia: a review. *British Journal of Community Nursing* **14**(10), 438–442.

Wood S (2008). Anatomy and physiology of pain. *Nursing Times*. 18th September.

World Health Organisation (1996). *WHO Guidelines: Cancer Pain*. 2nd edn. Geneva, World Health Organisation.

Early Warning Scoring Tools

8

INTRODUCTION

Vital signs are defined by Kozier et al. (2008, p. 337) as the 'physiological measures nurses record in clinical situations to assess the clinical status of patients on their care and to monitor for changes'. To address the importance of recording and monitoring patients' vital signs, scoring tools have been introduced into clinical practice. A physiological track and trigger system is a scoring tool that has been introduced into all acute National Health Service (NHS) trusts. The rationale for introducing a systematic tool was to provide an early warning of any potential problems with the patients' vital signs. There are several variations of the scoring tool that include 'Patients at Risk Score', 'Modified Early Warning Score' or 'Early Warning Scoring'. A National Early Warning Scoring (NEWS) system is due to be launched in 2011 (Pearce, 2011). For the purpose of this chapter, the assessment tool discussed will be referred to as the Early Warning Scoring (EWS) tool. In conjunction with the EWS, the 'Look, Listen and Feel' approach will also be discussed as a fundamental element in the assessment of recording and responding to the patient's vital signs.

LEARNING OUTCOMES

By the end of this chapter, you will be able to discuss the following:

❑ The principles of early warning scoring tools
❑ Performing and documenting the EWS

Vital Signs for Nurses: An Introduction to Clinical Observations, First Edition.
Joyce Smith and Rachel Roberts.
© 2011 Joyce Smith and Rachel Roberts. Published 2011 by Blackwell Publishing Ltd.

❑ The concept of Outreach and Medical Emergency Teams
❑ Government policies and guidelines

The EWS was developed at the James Padgett Hospital in Great Yarmouth as a tool that would identify patients who were becoming acutely ill. The National Institute for Health and Clinical Excellence (NICE, 2007), National Patient Safety Agency (NPSA, 2007a, 2007b) and the Department of Health (DH, 2009) all advocate the EWS as being integral to the early recognition that a patient is becoming acutely unwell.

THE PRINCIPLES OF THE EARLY WARNING SCORING SYSTEMS

The recommendation to implement the EWS system was based on concerns that patients were showing clinical signs of deterioration, but their physiological observations were not documented (McQuillan et al., 1998; Goldhill et al., 1999) or if their vital signs were documented, it was not recognised by clinical staff that there was a potential problem (National Confidential Enquiry into Patient Outcome and Death (NCEPOD), 2005). Taking and recording a patient's vital signs forms part of the patient's initial assessment. The purpose of assessment is to gain information and data that provide a baseline for clinical decision making. A constant theme that emerged from the previous research was that one important vital sign was no longer recorded as part of the patients' initial assessment. Despite the respiratory rate being identified as the most sensitive indicator that the patient is becoming acutely unwell, it was no longer recorded on the patient's observation charts (Kenward et al., 2001; NICE, 2007; NPSA, 2007). A qualitative study by Hogan (2006) found that the respiratory rate was the one parameter that was recorded less than 50% of the time. The reasons for not recording the respiratory rate included workload, skills training, decision making and a greater reliance on electronic devices. Watson (2006) suggests that applying the term 'basic' to clinical observations detracts from the value of recording a patient's vital signs.

The frequency of not accurately recording the patient's vital signs has been acknowledged as a national problem for nearly a decade and previously identified by the Department of Health

(DH) in the document 'Comprehensive Critical Care' (DH, 2000). A report by the National Confidential Enquiry into Patient Outcome and Death (NCEPOD, 2005) revealed that patients displayed prolonged physiological instability for more than 12 hours prior to being admitted to the intensive care unit (ICU). As a direct result of previous research that patients often receive suboptimal care (below an acceptable standard), the National Institute for Health and Clinical Excellence (NICE) produced Clinical Guideline 50, which recommended that all acute hospital settings introduce a track and trigger scoring systems and that physiological observations are performed on all patients on admission (NICE, 2007). In 2009, the Department of Health reinforced the introduction of NICE guidelines (DH, 2009).

The EWS tool has now been incorporated into the physiological observation charts within most acute hospital settings. However, you may find the EWS chart used as a separate tool or depending on your practice area, a different variation of the EWS tool in recording the patients' physiological observations. In the acute setting, it is now a recommendation that an EWS system be used to assess all patients on admission to hospital or at the initial assessment. At the time of admission, the initial assessment must include heart rate, respiratory rate, systolic blood pressure, level of consciousness, oxygen saturations and temperature (NICE, 2007).

It is the responsibility of individual healthcare organisations to decide if they include a track and trigger system or the EWS tool as part of their physiological observations chart. You may find that there are variations in the physiological parameters on the EWS tool and it is the responsibility of the acute trust to decide the parameters that are to be included (NICE, 2007). The EWS tool is based on the vital signs that healthcare staff are normally asked to perform and record daily (Table 8.1).

HOW TO COMPLETE AN EARLY WARNING SCORING CHART

It is recommended that only members of the healthcare team within an acute trust who have undertaken training should perform and record physiological observations (NICE, 2007; DH, 2009). Therefore, if you work in an acute trust, it is important that you are trained and assessed as *competent* to perform physiological observations. If a registered nurse delegates physiological observations to

Table 8.1 Sample of an Early Warning Scoring Tool. Reproduced under the terms of the Click-Use Licence.

Early Warning Scoring System

Score	3	2	1	0	1	2	3
Temperature		<35		35.0–38.3		≥38.4	
Systolic BP	<70	71–80	81–100	101–170	171–199	>200	
Pulse		<40	41–50	51–100	101–111	111–129	>130
Respiratory Rate		<8		8–18	19–22	23–29	>30
Consciousness Level AVPU		New agitation/confusion		**A** Alert	**V** Voice	**P** Pain	**U** Unresponsive
Urine		<30 ml/h For 2 h				>300 ml/hr for 2 h	

141

healthcare assistants, assistant practitioners or student nurses, they must ensure that they have completed their education and training through National Vocational Qualifications (NVQ) – for example, the NVQ unit CHS19 'Undertake Physiological Measurements' or an assessment introduced by the practice area. A registered nurse, who delegates physiological observations to a healthcare assistant, assistant practitioner or student nurse, is therefore responsible and accountable for the delegation (Nursing and Midwifery Council (NMC), 2008).

By adopting a systematic approach in completing the EWS tool, healthcare staff will provide important information that will inform the patient's assessment but also ensure that there are no omissions or failure to document each of the patient's baseline observations. As each vital sign is recorded, any deviations from the patient's normal parameters will create a score. On completion of the vital signs, the individual scores are added together and if the score is more than 3, a senior member of healthcare team needs to be informed or an escalation plan activated. If the score is less than 3, the patient's vital signs need to be monitored more frequently. On the sample EWS tool (Table 8.1), the baseline vital signs that are routinely performed on patients are each given a score from 0 to 3. On the left-hand side of the chart, you will see the observations that may be included (Refer Table 6.3), which include pulse, blood pressure, respiratory rate, temperature and consciousness level (**AVPU**) and urine output. There are EWS charts that also include the oxygen saturation.

Vital signs

Patients admitted to the theatre, a surgical or a respiratory ward may have their oxygen saturation measured as routine practice and all patients following an operation may have their oxygen saturations monitored. Therefore, oxygen saturation may also be routinely included as part of the EWS tool in recording the patient's vital signs. ICU and high dependency units (HDU) that care for acutely ill patients monitor the patient's oxygen saturations as an essential parameter when recording the patient's vital signs. Pulse oximetry is a simple non-invasive method of monitoring oxygen saturations by calculating the percentage of haemoglobin (Hb) that is saturated with oxygen (Jevon and Ewens, 2002). The pulse oximeter consists of a probe that is attached to the patient's finger or ear lobe; please note that the probe for the finger must not be used on the patient's ear. Special probes have been specifically designed for the ear to record oxygen saturations. To prevent the risk of cross-infection, the oximeter probe must be cleaned before being placed on the patient's finger or ear.

The position of the probe must also be changed at regular intervals, as leaving the probe for long periods of time may result in a pressure sore (Sadik et al., 2007). Once the probe is placed on the finger or ear, the pulse oximeter calculates the percentage of Hb saturated with oxygen at the peripheries. The pulse oximeter probe has two light-emitting diodes (you may have noticed a red light when you place the probe on the patient's finger or ear lobe) that transmit red and infrared light through body tissue. Light passes through the tissue and is sensed by the photodetector at the base of the probe. The normal range for the patient's oxygen saturation is between 95 and 100%; this is more commonly known and recorded as SpO_2 (Jevon and Ewens, 2002).

If you use a Dinamap® when monitoring the patient's vital signs, the equipment has the facility to record and display the patient's oxygen saturations. Pulse oximetry may be an important part of the physiological observations that are requested; therefore, it is important that the results are documented on the patient's chart. It is also necessary to understand that the pulse oximeter may produce false readings. For example, false nails, nail polish, shivering, cold hands and the lighting may all affect the reading (Please refer to Chapter 3). A new technique of using forehead sensors for taking pulse oximetry has been adopted in certain clinical areas. Forehead sensors are often applied when patients have poor peripheral perfusion, as arterial blood travelling from the heart reaches the head much sooner than it reached the hands.

Urine output

Urine output is an essential part of monitoring vital signs and several EWS tools include the urine output although NICE (2007) states that this is an optional parameter. An easy way to calculate the urine output is by knowing the patient's weight. If the patient's weight, for example, is 70 kg, you would calculate the urine output at the rate of 0.5 ml/kg to be 35 ml of urine/h. If it is not possible to weigh the patient or the patient's weight is not known, a guided measurement is that patients should pass at least 30 ml of urine per hour. If after 2 hours, the urine output is less than 60 ml or the patient passes excessive amounts of urine on completion of the EWS tool, senior members of the healthcare team need to be informed. Although the urine output may not always be included, the fluid balance chart is important in informing the assessment of the patient's vital signs. Recording an accurate fluid balance chart will provide data on a patient's hydration status and is normally completed over a 24-hour period. A positive balance is when the intake is greater than the output or a negative balance is when the output is greater than the input.

The consequences of not maintaining an accurate fluid balance chart may lead to delays in recognition that there is a potential problem. A fluid balance chart will provide signs and symptoms that you will be able to link to the patient's vital signs. For example, a reduced urine output may indicate dehydration that will be reflected by a drop in the patient's blood pressure or fluid overload that may result in pulmonary oedema and an increased respiratory rate.

By systematically completing the EWS tool you will be able to confirm that each vital sign is within the agreed parameters set by the trust or your employer. Always remember to complete all the vital signs identified on the EWS tool, as incorrect scores may potentially result in a lack of recognition that the patient is becoming unwell. Therefore, it is important that all the vital signs are recorded on the observation chart and documented in the patient's care plan.

On the EWS tool (Table 8.1), the patient's conscious level is assessed by the acronym *AVPU*. What do the letters A, V, P and U for assessing the level of consciousness mean?

A – (Alert) Conscious, alert, eyes open, orientated and able to answer questions.

V – (Responds to Voice) Not Alert, semiconscious and may have their eyes closed. On hearing a voice will respond when roused.

P – (Responds only to pain) only moves or groans in response to painful stimuli administered by the doctor or registered nurse. If a patient is only responding to pain, urgent referral is required as P equates to a score of 8 on the Glasgow Coma Scale. The patient's airway is at risk.

U – (Unconscious) No response to voice or painful stimuli.

When using a manual sphygmomanometer to record the blood pressure, remember that you need to calculate the mean arterial pressure. For example, if the blood pressure is 180/60, add the systolic 180 and double the diastolic, that is, $60 + 60 = 120$ ($180 + 120 = 300$); the total is 300; divide it by 3 ($300 \div 3 = 100$); therefore, the mean arterial pressure is 100. Alternatively, if the blood pressure is 180/60, take 60 away from 180, that is, ($180 - 60 = 120$), divide 120 by 3 ($120 \div 3 = 40$), add the 40 to the diastolic ($40 + 60 = 100$) and the mean arterial pressure is 100.

Applying a systematic approach in performing the patient's vital signs and calculating the score for each of the physiological observations that may have deviated from the set parameters will provide the healthcare team with important information for any further action (Simpson, 2006). The importance of accurately recording the EWS and how nurses interpret the scores has been the focus of previous studies by Oakey and Slade (2006) and Smith and Oakey (2006), who revealed that the EWS was not always documented correctly often due to the business of the ward. Equally, a significant number of EWS tools had incorrect scores. A recent snapshot survey completed by 830 visitors to www.nursingtimes.net highlighted that nurses are failing to monitor a patient's vital signs. The consequence of not monitoring the patient's vital signs is lack of recognition of the patient deteriorating (Lomas and West, 2009a).

The EWS tool is an integral part of the assessment and recording of the patient's vital signs; equally importantly, the tool should be used in line with the nurse's knowledge and skills. It is an important part of the healthcare professionals' role in performing and recording physiological observations to be assessed as competent (NICE, 2007). Healthcare professionals can make a difference to the safety of patients by identifying the clinical changes to the patients' vital signs and informing senior members of the healthcare team (NPSA, 2007). The important information you provide to the healthcare team will initiate a systematic approach to the clinical interventions required. An Early Warning Scoring tool including the Referral and Escalation System (EWSRE) or flow chart has been devised and implemented in several trusts (Fig. 8.1). Linking the EWS score to a graded response or escalation chart will result in a systematic approach to the management of an acutely ill patient (Day and Oldroyd, 2010).

The systematic approach outlined in the flow chart ensures that appropriate action is taken. In recognition of the suboptimal care that patients may receive, the Department of Health, in their document 'Comprehensive Critical Care' (2000), made recommendations for the development and introduction of *Outreach Teams or Medical Emergency Teams* that are reinforced by NICE (2007).

THE CONCEPT OF OUTREACH AND MEDICAL EMERGENCY TEAMS

Recommendations by the Department of Health (2000) and the NICE (2007) to introduce outreach or medical emergency teams were aimed not only at supporting patients who are becoming acutely ill but also at educating and developing the clinical skills necessary for nursing staff to care for acutely ill patients. By identifying patients who are becoming acutely unwell, the Outreach or Medical Emergency Team may prevent further deterioration or a timely admission to a HDU or an ICU. The recommendations for developing Outreach or Medical Emergency Teams have not been implemented in all trusts (Fig. 8.2).

Practice point 8.1

Look at the observation chart below.

Q1. Work out the EWS score from Table 8.1
Q2. Are there any observations that are not recorded?
Q3. Have you noticed if there are any trends with the recorded observations?
Q4. Does the chart also provide information on what is happening to the patient's physiological observations that have previously been documented?
Q5. What clinical action should be taken?

Early Warning Scoring

The pennine Acute Hospitals **NHS**
NHS Trust

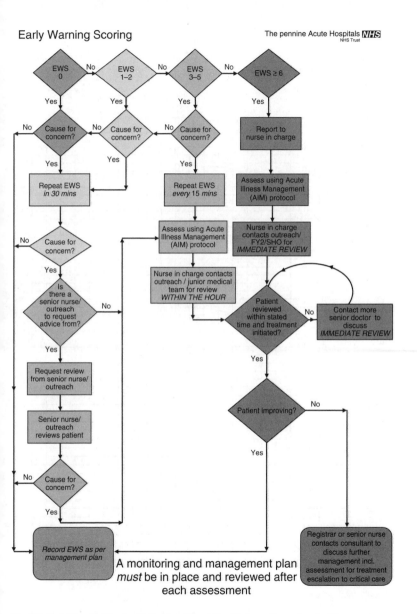

Fig. 8.1 Early Warning Scoring Referral and Escalation System. Reproduced with permission from Pennine Acute Hospitals NHS Trust.

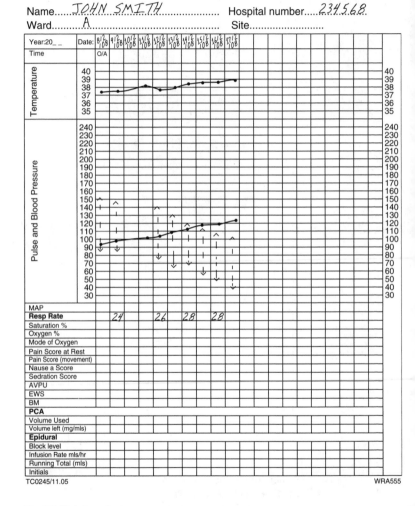

Fig. 8.2 Vital signs chart.

After completing the practice point, you may have noticed from this chart that it shows a trend in the physiological observations of the patient. For example, there is a continuous rise in the respiratory rate and the heart rate; however, the blood pressure is continuously on a downward trend.

The sign of the blood pressure going down and the heart rate rising is often called the seagull or pigeon sign. Imagine that the arrows of the systolic BP ↑ represent the wings of a bird and the pulse represents the fact that birds always 'poo' downwards. If you see the pulse above the wings of the bird, it is a warning that your patient is becoming critically unwell and in the poo!

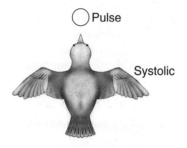

It is clear from the observation chart that the pigeon sign is already evident and your patient is becoming acutely unwell. It is important not only to document the clinical vital signs of the patient and calculate the score accurately but also to recognise that there is a *trend* in the vital signs chart and that senior members of the healthcare team need to be informed. The National Patient Safety Agency (NPSA), following an analysis of 576 deaths over a period of 1 year in 2005, reported that 11% ($n = 66$) of the deaths were a result of the deterioration not being recognised or acted upon. Although the NPSA recognised from the findings that there are complex issues, three themes emerged – no observations taken for a prolonged period of time and therefore changes in the patient's observations not detected; no recognition of the importance of the patient's deterioration; and no action taken other than the actual recording of the vital signs, often resulting in a delay in receiving medical attention. Poor record keeping has legal and professional consequences for healthcare staff (Griffith and Tengnah, 2010). Equally importantly, calculating EWS incorrectly and not applying basic visual observations were identified as issues that contributed to a lack of recognition that a patient may have clinical signs of deteriorating (NPSA, 2007).

A retrospective study by Oakey and Slade (2006) has indicated that there is often no interpretation or recognition that the patient is becoming acutely unwell. The majority of healthcare settings record the patients' vital signs on handwritten charts and manually calculate the EWS score. However, in several acute hospital trusts, handheld computers are being piloted or introduced as a way of inputting patient observations. The handheld computer then calculates the individual EWS, and in certain types of handheld computers, the score is plotted against a series of indicators to show whether the patient's condition is deteriorating (Tweddell, 2008). A study by Mohammed et al. (2009) comparing paper-based versus handheld electronic methods of calculating the EWS scores found that handheld computers improved the accuracy of nursing staff calculations.

By contrast, questions have been raised regarding the use of technology when undertaking vital signs – for example, a Dinamap or a pulse oximeter. Lomas and West (2009b) discussed the potential concerns of automated technology to monitor vital signs and suggested that there is a potential to deskill nursing staff. Boulanger and Toghill (2009) question the value of using automated machines, for example, a Dinamap, when monitoring patient's vital signs is perceived by healthcare staff as a clinical task and not as an essential part of ensuring safer patient outcomes. Technology is now an important part of care delivery, but healthcare professionals must prove their competence when using electronic equipment. According to Preston and Flynn (2010), it is not only having the competence in using electronic monitoring devices that is crucial but also having the knowledge and skills to interpret the physiological responses that are activated when a patient shows signs of clinical deterioration. Previously, nursing staff recorded the patients' vital signs, but the interpretation was not an expected part of their remit (Watson, 2006); however, there is now an expectation that nursing staff have the knowledge and skills to interpret the patients' vital signs.

Practice point 8.2

Mrs Jones has been admitted to the medical ward following a chest infection. On admission, she has a respiratory rate of 18, pulse 120 and her blood pressure is 130/70, and temperature is 37.7. She is alert but feels very poorly. The following day, her respiratory rate is 22, pulse is 120, blood pressure is 110/70 and her temperature is 37.9. At 2 pm when you complete her observations, the respiratory rate is 28, pulse 125, temperature 38, oxygen saturations 90% and blood pressure 102/65 and she also appears to be more confused.

Q1. What is Mrs Jones' latest EWS according to Table 6.3?
Q2. What are the clinical signs of deterioration in relation to Mrs Jones?
Q3. What action do you need to take as a result of her physiological observations?

LOOK, LISTEN AND FEEL WHEN USING THE EWS

It is important that the 'Look, Listen and Feel' systematic approach is applied in the EWS assessment of a patient (Watson, 2006).

Look at the patient and observe for signs of pale or peripherally cyanosed skin. Sometimes the skin can be pink and flushed. Is the breathing pattern regular or irregular, slow or fast and is the patient using the accessory muscles (shoulders or stomach muscles) to help them breathe? (Jevon and Ewens, 2001) Does the patient also appear agitated or confused indicating a change in level of consciousness?

Listen to the patients when they respond to your questions. Note how the patients respond to the questions. Do they sound confused or are they orientated and replying appropriately? Do you hear any noises that are abnormal – for example, gurgling or wheezing? Are you concerned? Is the electronic monitoring device alarming? What action do you need to take as a result of your concerns?

Feel the patient's skin and note whether it feels cool, cold, clammy or hot and sweating. Is the manual pulse regular, or weak, thready or is it bounding and fast?

A systematic approach to performing physiological observations including the look, listen and feel approach will provide valuable information to inform senior members of the healthcare team of the patients' condition.

In March 2009, the Department of Health devised a framework of competencies for healthcare staff in recognising and responding to acutely ill patients in hospital. The framework is in response to concerns that the early recognition and response to signs of deterioration in adult patients was often delayed. The framework supports the implementation of the NICE (2007) clinical guideline, which recommends that all members of the multidisciplinary team be competent in performing, recording, interpreting and responding to a patient's physiological observations. The competencies are based on the 'Chain of Response' (Fig. 8.3). The six chains are *non-clinical staff* (this may include the patient or visitor), *recorder* (the person who takes the physiological measurements), *recogniser* (the person who interprets the measurements and information), *primary responder* (initiates clinical measurements and clinical management plan), *secondary responder* (who attends the patients if they fail to respond) *and tertiary responder* (who is competent to assess critically ill patients). The ability to recognise signs of deterioration in the patient and respond is a key element in all six chains that reinforces the importance of communication and handover (DH, 2009, p. 7). Although the competencies target hospital-based staff, they may also be adapted and used in other settings.

Each link in the chain of response relates to your knowledge and skills in recording, recognising and including action as a primary responder. The registered nurse is identified as the recogniser or responder. Experienced members of the healthcare team who have undertaken further training or are based in a critical care area will possess the competencies required of the secondary and tertiary responders to assess critically ill patients. Underpinning the chain of response is the recommendation that multidisciplinary staff

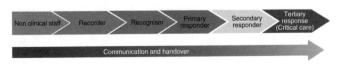

Fig. 8.3 'Chain of Response' (DH, 2008). Reproduced under the terms of the Click-Use Licence.

have successfully been assessed as competent in performing physiological observations and by attending recognised courses – for example, Basic Life Support (BLS), Acute Life Threatening Events Recognition and Treatment (ALERT), Intermediate Life Support (ILS) or the Acute Illness Management (AIM) course (DH, 2009).

CONCLUSION

In this chapter, we have identified that the EWS system is a valuable tool for recognising and responding to patients who are becoming acutely unwell. Every patient is an individual and may not, in certain circumstances, trigger a score; therefore, observational and experiential skills of the look, listen and feel approach provide a valuable tool when performing the patient's assessment. Accurate documentation and effective communication are necessary to ensure a timely multidisciplinary team approach when caring for acutely ill patients. Early recognition and treatment of the patient's vital signs that are outside of the normal parameters may prevent patients from becoming acutely unwell or identify timely recognition of deterioration (NICE, 2007; NPSA, 2007; DH, 2009).

REFERENCES

Boulanger C and Toghill M (2009). How to measure and record vital signs to ensure detection of deteriorating patients. *Nursing Times* **105**(47), 10–12.

Day A and Oldroyd C (2010). The use of early warning scores in the emergency department. *Journal of Emergency Nursing* **36**(2), 154–155.

Department of Health (DH) (2000). *Comprehensive Critical Care: A Review of Adult Critical Care Services*. London, The Stationery Office.

Department of Health (2008). Competencies for recognising and responding to acutely ill patients in hospital. *Consultation Document*. Published to DH website, in electronic PDF format only. http://www.dh.gov.uk/publications.

Department of Health (DH) (2009). *Competencies for Recognising and Responding to Acutely Ill Patients in Hospital*. http://www.dh.gov.uk/publications.

Goldhill DA, White SA, and Sumner A (1999). Physiological values and procedures in the 24h before ICU admission from the ward. *Anaesthesia* **54**, 529–534.

Griffith R and Tengnah C (2010). *Law and Professional Issues in Nursing*. 2nd edn. Exeter, Learning Matters Ltd.

Hogan J (2006). Why don't nurses monitor the respiratory rates of patients? *British Journal of Nursing* **15**(9), 489–492.

Jevon P and Ewens B (2001). Assessment of a breathless patient. *Nursing Standard* **15**(16), 48–53.

Jevon P and Ewens B (2002). *Monitoring the Critically Ill Patient*. Oxford, Blackwell Publishing Ltd.

Kenward G, Castle N, and Hodgetts T (2001). Time to put the R back in TPR. *Nursing Times* **97**(40), 32–33.

Kozier B, Glencora E, Berman A, Snyder S, Lake R, and Harvey S (2008). *Fundamentals of Nursing Concepts, Process and Practice*. London, Pearson Education.

Lomas C and West D (2009a). Poor observation skills are risking patients' lives. *Nursing Times* http://www.nursingtimes.net/5007194article. [Accessed 15th May 2010].

Lomas C and West D (2009b). Skills lost as automation takes over. *Nursing Times* **105**(40), 2–3.

McQuillan P, Pilkington A, Allan A et al. (1998). Confidential inquiry into quality of care before admission to intensive care. *British Medical Journal* **316**, 1853–1858.

Mohammed MA, Hayton R, Clements G, Smith G, and Prytherch D (2009). Improving accuracy and efficiency of early warning scores in acute care. *British Journal of Nursing* **18**(1), 18–24.

National Confidential Enquiry into Patient Outcome and Death (NCEPOD) (2005). *An Acute Problem?* www.ncepod.org.uk [Accessed 12th March 2008].

National Institute for Health and Clinical Excellence (NICE) (2007). *Acutely Ill Patients in Hospital: Recognition and Response to Acute Illness in Adults in Hospital*. Guideline 50. London, NICE.

National Patient Safety Agency (NPSA) (2007a). *Recognising and Responding Appropriately to Early Signs of Deterioration in Hospitalised Patients*. London. http//tinyurl.com/yk8qbx5 [Accessed 26th March 20010].

National Patient Safety Agency (NPSA) (2007b). *Safer care for the acutely ill patient: learning from serious incidents*. London. http://www.nrls.npsa.nhs.uk/resources/?entryid45=59828 [Accessed 26th March 2010].

Nursing and Midwifery Council (2008). The Code. *Standards of Conduct, Performance and Ethics for Nurses and Midwives*. London, NMC. www.nmc.org.uk [Accessed 12th April 2009].

Oakey RJ, Slade V (2006). Physiological observation track and trigger system. *Nursing Standard* **27**, 48–54.

Pearce L (2011). *Taking a Critical Role*. London, RCN Publishing Company Ltd.

Preston R and Flynn D (2010). Observations in acute care: evidence-based approach to patient safety. *British Journal of Nursing* **19**(7), 442–447.

Sadik R, Walker C, and Elliott D (2007). Respiration and circulation. In: *Foundations of Nursing Practice Leading the Way*, Hogston R and Marjoram BA (eds). London, Palgrave Macmillan.

Simpson H (2006). Respiratory assessment. *British Journal of Nursing* **15**(9), 484–488.

Smith AF and Oakey RJ (2006). Incidence and significance of errors in a patient 'track and trigger' system during an epidemic of Legionnaires disease: retrospective case note analysis. *Anaesthesia* **61**(3), 222–228.

Tweddell L (2008). Computer power on the wards. *Nursing Times* **104**(38), 18–19.

Watson D (2006). The impact of accurate patient assessment on quality of care. *Nursing Times* **102**(6), 34.

Communication

9

INTRODUCTION

Previous chapters have focused on the different components of vital signs monitoring. However, being able to perform vital signs in the clinical arena brings the added responsibility of recognising the significance of improving or deteriorating observations and the need to communicate it to the rest of the clinical team. Timely and effective communication will ensure that patients who are at risk of further clinical deterioration will receive the appropriate clinical intervention.

The daily activity of performing vital signs on patients and reporting the readings, in a timely manner, is as important as having the skills to perform these observations. Communicating to colleagues regarding clinical care and activities undertaken is expressed through verbal dialogue as well as by recording activities in the care plans and recording information on the physiological charts.

LEARNING OUTCOMES

By the end of this chapter, you will be able to discuss the following:

❑ The ways in which patients and staff communicate with each other
❑ The importance of timely communication in relation to deteriorating clinical observations
❑ Reporting findings

Vital Signs for Nurses: An Introduction to Clinical Observations, First Edition.
Joyce Smith and Rachel Roberts.
© 2011 Joyce Smith and Rachel Roberts. Published 2011 by Blackwell Publishing Ltd.

❏ The need for team work to promote the best care for the patient
❏ The role of communication tools

WAYS IN WHICH PATIENTS AND STAFF COMMUNICATE WITH EACH OTHER

The ability to communicate effectively with patients and colleagues is a vital part of day-to-day activity. In its most basic form, communication has three elements: sender, message and receiver (Ellis et al., 2006).

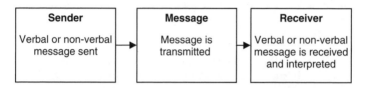

Human beings send messages to each other verbally and non-verbally. These messages are transmitted using verbal and non-verbal communication pathways. The message is then received and processed. The receiver will then interpret the information and may communicate a response and feedback to the sender.

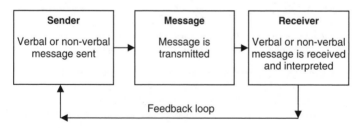

Communication is not just about talking; it is also about how the multiprofessional team communicates using different styles. Staff may communicate verbally through face-to-face conversations or via telephone conversations. Non-verbal communication can be interpreted by looking at the signs and signals of a person's behaviour, such as facial expressions and posture. Written and non-verbal communication can be made through the computer, using email or through text messaging on mobile phones. Nurses should be aware that electronic records such as texts, email or computer-held information apply to the principles of good record keeping according to the Nursing and Midwifery Council (NMC, 2009) guidelines. Communication skills are essential for building up therapeutic relationships with patients. On a daily basis, clinical staff will use their interpersonal skills to be able to gather information, question, answer and listen to the patient and other healthcare colleagues (Hamilton and Martin, 2007). Communication is very important to patients, as they rely on the nurse for honest and sensitive explanation, reassurance and support in the provision of the care they receive.

There are many barriers to effectively getting a message understood. The cyclical diagram in Fig. 9.1 identifies a few of the potential barriers. Barriers can be created either by the sender or by the receiver. If the sender is using language and jargon that this not understood by the receiver, then the message will not be recognized or acted on. If the sender sends a message in a rush (e.g. texting a message to the wrong person), it could result in misunderstandings.

Practice point 9.1

You have been asked to review Mr and Mrs Collins at their home. Mr Collins was recently diagnosed with Alzheimer's disease but is currently suffering from a community-acquired chest infection.

(a) Identify the potential barriers you need to consider when gaining consent to taking his blood pressure, pulse, respiration and temperature.
(b) What communication strategies can you use to break down these potential barriers?

Patients who come to the healthcare centre or hospital will have their own preconceived ideas and expectations about what will happen. Their anxiety and fear may also inhibit their ability to effectively receive and respond to questions or information being relayed. Patients have their own ideas about what a nurse or

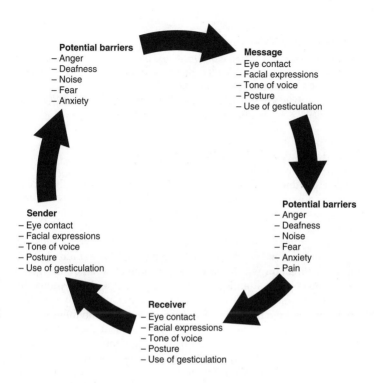

Potential barriers
– Anger
– Deafness
– Noise
– Fear
– Anxiety

Message
– Eye contact
– Facial expressions
– Tone of voice
– Posture
– Use of gesticulation

Sender
– Eye contact
– Facial expressions
– Tone of voice
– Posture
– Use of gesticulation

Potential barriers
– Anger
– Deafness
– Noise
– Fear
– Anxiety
– Pain

Receiver
– Eye contact
– Facial expressions
– Tone of voice
– Posture
– Use of gesticulation

Fig. 9.1 How to send the right message – beware of barriers.

doctor does and this form of stereotyping can lead to problems in communication. Equally importantly, healthcare professionals may make stereotypical judgements about patients because of their own belief systems. Belief systems, although personal, must not inhibit professional behaviour and conduct when dealing with patients. Staff are encouraged to use reflection (Chapter 13) about their conduct and behaviours to avoid bias and prejudice when performing care and treatment for patients. Lack of privacy in a noisy hospital ward can also inhibit communication. Some patients may be deaf and have difficulty in hearing you and may rely on their visual systems to decipher messages.

Practice point 9.2

Think about the last patient on whom you performed clinical observations. How did your non-verbal and verbal communication affect your approach towards the patient in gaining consent for you to perform them? Compare your thoughts and ideas when reading the following look, listen and feel section.

USING THE LOOK, LISTEN AND FEEL APPROACH IN COMMUNICATION

When commencing a clinical shift, it is useful to walk down the ward and take a *look* around and make a mental note of the activities that are happening at the patient's bedside. By doing this, you can begin to use your visual and listening skills to interpret how the patients and staff feel at that time as well as gain a sense of what sort of mood people are in. It is amazing how a smile or a nod in their direction will bring about a response. Maintaining good eye contact gains attention and may be the icebreaker required to start a conversation with colleagues or patients. When approaching the patients, give them good eye contact and focus on them so that they know that you are genuinely interested in them. Take the time to ask them how they are. In this way, you are giving them an opportunity to tell you how they are feeling at that time. They may tell you that they are fine or that they are in pain or they may not choose to respond at all. *Listen* and look for a response before explaining to them that you would like to perform their clinical observations.

Maintaining good eye contact as well as providing information about the rationale of why you wish to perform the observations will increase the likelihood that the patients will give consent. They may demonstrate their consent to have their clinical observations performed by nodding, holding out their arm for you to put on the BP cuff or they may simply state 'OK, that's fine'.

Sometimes, the patient will watch you quietly as you perform vital signs monitoring or they may continue to carry on the conversation. This can cause some difficulties when you are trying to count the respiratory rate and listen to them at the same time, causing you to lose count! A useful way to limit the amount of

Table 9.1 Elements of SOLER.

S	*Sit* squarely in relation to the patient
O	*Open* position (no closed, folded arms)
L	*Lean* slightly towards the patient
E	*Eye* contact with the patient (but do not continuously stare)
R	*Relax*

chatter while you count is to take the manual pulse at the same time. People naturally realise that you will be counting and will be quiet for this. Keep your fingers on the pulse until you have also been able to count the respiration rate correctly. You can then tell the patient what the readings are if they are interested in knowing.

Egan (2002) recommends the acronym SOLER to promote effective and active listening skills. Table 9.1 gives an outline of each element of SOLER.

Using SOLER will encourage you to focus on the patient. Good eye contact demonstrates to the patients that you are giving them your undivided attention and will increase your ability to listen effectively. Listening also involves the ability to be silent and at times it is appropriate to be quiet and allow silence to occur. Silence allows both patient and staff time to reflect upon the conversation and provide thinking time before speaking again. Silence also allows time to think about verbal and non-verbal behaviour and mannerisms during interaction.

THE IMPORTANCE OF TIMELY COMMUNICATION IN RELATION TO DETERIORATING CLINICAL OBSERVATIONS

Within each NHS trust, the use of track and trigger systems for the monitoring of physiological observations of the acutely ill patient is expected (NICE, 2007; 2008). Abnormal physiological observations must be reported as soon as possible to the person in charge or to the person who has delegated you this role. This has been emphasised within the NICE guidance where it states as follows:

> Physiological measurements should be recorded and acted on by staff who have been trained to undertake these procedures and understand their clinical relevance.

(NICE, 2007, p. 8)

Practice point 9.3

It is 08.00 am and you have just completed the observations on Mrs Peters, a first day post-op patient, following surgery for removal of gallstones (cholecystectomy). Mrs Peters says that she feels nauseated and is getting a lot of pain around the surgical wound site. The patient's current observations are RR 24, saturations 90%, HR 115, BP 100/50, and temperature 38.1°C. Would these observations cause concern to you?

What communication systems and strategies will you use to address your concerns to other members of the multidisciplinary team?

An effective way to raise your concerns to colleagues is to use the communication framework of SBAR developed by Kaiser Permanente (Institute for Health Improvement (IHI), 2008). Ideally, talk to members of the team face to face and tell them about the **Situation** of the patient, their clinical **Background**, their current clinical **Assessment** and **Recommendations**. If you take the first letter of each bolded word, it makes the acronym **SBAR**. You may find this adapted SBAR communication framework (see Tables 9.2 and 9.3) useful to gather your thoughts about how to convey the information more effectively.

According to Murray et al. (2006), communication skills are the essence of any interaction, whether it is personal, professional, social or otherwise, but the structure must be present to build up the likelihood of effective interaction.

Table 9.2 Adapted SBAR communication tool.

S = Situation	Explain who you are and where you are calling from Explain what the purpose of the conversation is
B = Background	Explain recent, relevant history and current circumstances
A = Assessment	Explain what assessment has been carried out and what the current problem is
R = Recommendation	Explain what you specifically want or need from the person you are calling

Table 9.3 Adapted SBAR framework to report to concerns about the physiological observations of Mrs Peters in Practice point 9.2.

Situation	'Hello Staff Nurse. I am concerned about Mrs Peters. She is first day post op and I have just completed her observations. Her vital signs are: RR = 24 HR = 115 BP = 100/50 Temperature = 38.1°C I am concerned because her Track and Trigger score is Her heart rate is faster than before and her BP has dropped from previous and she has spiked a temperature'
Background	**Patient's mental state**: 'Mrs Peters is alert, but is feeling nauseous. She says she has severe pain' **Skin colour**: 'Mrs Peters is looking very pale and her hands and arm felt cold to touch when I took her BP' **The patient is/is not on oxygen**: 'Mrs Peters has oxygen via the nasal cannula at 4 litres per minute and her saturations are currently reading 90%, but previously were reading 98%'
Assessment	**I think the problem is:** 'her pain from her surgical site. Her abdomen does look swollen and she has got a temperature. I am not sure what the underlying cause is but she has definitely deteriorated'
Recommendation	**I suggest/request:** 'Staff Nurse, please can you come and see Mrs Peters now and review her. I have brought you the prescription sheet to review her painkillers' **Are any test needed:** 'Mrs Peters is looking very pale, maybe she is anaemic. Shall I take blood tests, such as a FBC and Clotting?' **Change in treatment is ordered by Staff Nurse**: 'How often do you want me to record Mrs Peters' observations' 'Thank you for giving her some pain killers and anti-emetic. I'll recheck Mrs Peter's observations in 20 minutes and reassess her track and trigger and pain score to see if the treatment is working' 'Staff Nurse, I'll keep you informed'

Hamilton and Martin (2007) recommends an alternative five-point communication structured framework when dealing with patients. These are given below in the figure.

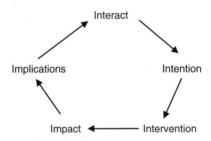

First, interact with the patient by talking to them and establishing good eye contact. In this way, you can use visual information as well as verbal information to ascertain how the patient is feeling. During the conversation, tell the patient what your intentions are and the reasons for why the intervention is required. Once consent is obtained, carry out the clinical intervention. Assess the impact of the interventions and then evaluate the implications and report the results to senior colleagues.

REPORTING FINDINGS

There are various frameworks that can be used to communicate to colleagues the results of vital signs. It is important that you are familiar with the hospital policy and procedures for reporting your findings. As previously discussed, it is important to verbally inform the nurse in charge as soon as possible, but another aspect to reporting your findings is to record accurately the results on the clinical observations charts. This information can also be reinforced when recorded in the care plan as part of good record keeping practices (refer to Chapter 12).

THE NEED FOR TEAM WORK TO PROMOTE BEST CARE FOR THE PATIENT

Staff should be aware of the importance of effective teamwork to promote the best care for the patient (Atwal, 2007). A lack of teamwork will lead to delays in the provision of appropriate patient care and impact on the quality of care provided. It is thought that between 70 and 80% of healthcare errors are caused by human factors related to poor team communication and understanding (Schaefer et al., 1994). An effective team will function properly only if each member is 'competent to collaborate' (Barr, 1998).

It is possible that in both the community and the acute setting, healthcare assistants will have been delegated a group of patients to care for by the registered nurse and therefore must be involved in the multidisciplinary meetings or ward rounds. Treating colleagues within the team and patients with dignity and respect will reduce the amount of challenging conversations and reduce conflicts of interest for patients and staff. Being self-aware of your behaviour, persona and personal beliefs also enhances your ability to understand other points of view, as well as empowering you to be less emotional or prejudiced in your responses and more objective. You can learn more about self-awareness in Chapter 14. Showing respect to another person during interaction and communication during ward rounds will promote and facilitate common ground to find solutions for better patient care.

CONCLUSION

This chapter has discussed how important communication is between patients and staff. Highlighted in this chapter are the communication tools of SOLER and SBAR that may be adopted by staff to encourage effective ways of communication when using EWS and the escalation policy for preventing deterioration of patients. Good communication strategies include written records as well as verbal dialogue. Within health care, teamwork is essential between the multidisciplinary teams to ensure that patients get the right care, at the right time, by the right person and in the right place.

REFERENCES

Atwal A (2007). The importance of the multidisciplinary team. *British Journal of Healthcare Assistants* **1**(9), 425–428.

Barr H (1998). Competent to collaborate: towards a competency-based model for interprofessional education. *Journal of Interprofessional Care* **12**(2), 181–188.

Egan G (2002). *The Skilled Helper: A Problem Management and Opportunity Approach to Helping*. Cambridge, Thomson Brooks/Cole.

Ellis RB, Gates B and Kenworthy N (2006). *Interpersonal Communication in Nursing Theory and Practice*. 2nd edn. Philadelphia, Churchill Livingstone.

Hamilton S and Martin DJ (2007). A framework for effective communication skills. *Nursing Times* **103**(48), 30–31.

Institute for Health Improvement (2008). www.ihi.org.

Murray K et al. (2006). Effective communication and its delivery in midwifery practice. *The Practicing Midwife* **9**(4), 24–26.

National Institute for Health and Clinical Excellence (NICE) (2007). *Acutely Ill Patients in Hospital. Recognition of and Response to Acute Illness in Adults in Hospitals*. London, NICE.

National Institute for Health and Clinical Excellence (NICE) (2008). *Competencies for Recognising and Responding to Acutely Ill Patients*. London, NICE.

Nursing and Midwifery Council (2009). *Guidance for Nurses and Midwives*. www.nmc.org?. Record Keeping.

Schaefer HG, Helreich RL, and Scheideggar D (1994). Human factors and safety in emergency medicine. *Resuscitation* **28**, 221–225.

Nutrition

10

INTRODUCTION

Nutrition is the study of nutrients and how the body processes the nutrients within the body. Nutrients are substances in foods required by the body for energy, growth, repair and restoration of cells and tissues (Grodner et al., 2004).

Eating and drinking are essential for living. According to the Department of Health (DH, 2007, p. 2), 'Good nutrition and hydration and enjoyable mealtimes can dramatically improve the health and well being of older people'. It should be viewed as a central component of patient care (O'Regan, 2009). For many people in residential care, mealtimes are the highlight of the day (DH, 2007) and the same can be said for patients in hospital.

Good clinical observations are required to ensure that patients are receiving good nutritional intake and adequate hydration. It is recognised that healthy eating and enjoyable mealtimes may improve the general health and well-being of people, as well as improving the immune system so that the body can fight illness. Being healthy will also reduce a person's length of stay in hospital and increase post-operative recovery (DH, 2007).

It is estimated that malnutrition costs the United Kingdom £7.3 billion a year. Out of every 10 people admitted to the hospital, 6 of them are at risk of becoming malnourished or deteriorating while in hospital (British Association for Parenteral and Enteral Nutrition (BAPEN), 2003, 2006). Therefore, nutrition has become a

Vital Signs for Nurses: An Introduction to Clinical Observations, First Edition.
Joyce Smith and Rachel Roberts.
© 2011 Joyce Smith and Rachel Roberts. Published 2011 by Blackwell Publishing Ltd.

high priority within health care and should be viewed as equally important to a person receiving medications (DH, 2007).

LEARNING OUTCOMES

By the end of this chapter, you will be able to discuss the following:

❑ The role of the gastrointestinal tract in the body
❑ The effects of poor nutrition on health and recovery of patients
❑ The definition of malnutrition
❑ The role of nutritional screening using the look, listen and feel approach
❑ The role of nutritional assessments tools (MUST tool)
❑ The different routes through which nutrition can be provided (oral, enteral and parenteral)
❑ The role of the unqualified nurse in monitoring and reporting the nutritional intake of patients

THE ROLE OF THE GASTROINTESTINAL (GI) TRACT IN THE BODY

The gastrointestinal (GI) tract is made up of the mouth, oesophagus, stomach and intestines, which extends from the mouth to the anus. The accessory digestive glands include the salivary glands, pancreas, liver and gall bladder. To review the anatomy of the GI tract, see Fig. 10.1.

Digestion

When we eat food, the first step in the process of breaking it down into fuel is to chew it in the mouth. The teeth break the food into smaller portions that are mixed with saliva. Saliva is made up of digestive enzymes. Once we have broken the food down into small enough pieces, we swallow it. The swallowed food travels down the oesophagus and the strong muscles in the oesophagus squeeze it down the 25-cm pipe until it reaches the stomach (Waugh and Grant, 2001).

Once the food is in the stomach, more digestive enzymes and hydrochloric acid are added to continue the process of breaking down the food into small particles to be absorbed through the large and small intestines. The food remains in the stomach for a few

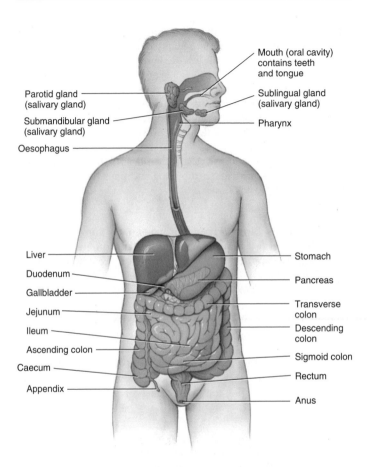

Fig. 10.1 Gastrointestinal tract. Reprinted with permission of John Wiley and Sons Inc.

hours. During these few hours, small amounts of food are then transported to the duodenum via the sphincter of Oddi.

In the duodenum, the gall bladder adds *bile* to the semi-digested mixture as well as *digestive enzymes* from the pancreas to further break the food down into glucose. Some of the glucose is used for any immediate fuel needs of the cells and tissues. The surplus glucose is sent to the liver to be stored as glycogen and once the glycogen stores in the liver are full, any remaining glucose will be turned into fat and stored around the organs and subcutaneous tissues.

As the digesting food travels down the small and large intestines bowels, a lot of water also is reabsorbed into the body, which then leaves digestive waste, commonly known as *faeces*. Strong bowel muscles squeeze the faeces along the bowel and mucous also helps to lubricate and ease the passage until it reaches the rectum. Faeces is stored here until the muscles spasm and send the message to the brain to relax the muscles of the anus and pass the faeces out of the body (Waugh and Grant, 2001).

FOOD GROUPS

The body needs carbohydrates, proteins, fats, fibre, water, vitamins and minerals within the body for many different functions (Smith and Watson, 2006). We shall have a more detailed look at each of these.

Carbohydrates

Carbohydrates are made up of carbon, oxygen and hydrogen and are essential for the production of heat and energy. Carbohydrates are made up of starch and sugar. Starch and sugar are broken down by the digestive system into glucose. Glucose is the primary resource for fuel for the body to create energy. Different examples of carbohydrates are potatoes, rice, oats, bread and pasta.

Fats

Fats are required to create heat and energy. Fats are stored around adipose tissues and major organs to provide protection and cushioning. Fats will be turned into glucose and converted into fuel for the body if there is a lack of carbohydrates or proteins in the body. The recommended amount of fat in diet should be less than 35% of total energy intake. Different examples of fats include butter, full fat milk, olive oil, cream and cheese.

Fibre

Fibre is essential to help with the elimination of waste (faeces) and in maintaining the amount of GI bacteria to a minimum. Fibre speeds up the time it takes for food to travel through the small and large intestines before it is excreted. Lack of fibre can slow down the time it takes for food to travel through the small and large intestines and can lead to problems such as constipation and bowel cancer. If the GI bacteria have been allowed to increase because of poor GI peristalsis, a person can then become unwell because the high levels of GI bacteria make them feel poorly. Different examples of fibre include pulses, cereals, oats, beans and green vegetables such as broccoli and cabbage.

Proteins
Proteins are commonly known as the *building blocks* of life. Proteins are required by the body to make different types of cells and tissues. Proteins are broken down by the body into amino acids. The body has a core requirement of 20 amino acids that can be used as central ingredients to make up more cells and tissues for the body. Proteins are made up of hydrogen, carbon, oxygen and nitrogen. When the GI tract breaks down protein, it will use the hydrogen, carbon and oxygen but not nitrogen, as it is toxic to the body. Nitrogen is disposed of by the body in the form of urine. Different examples of proteins include chicken, beef, pork, lamb, cheese and beans.

Water
Water is crucial for life and the human being is made up of two-thirds of water. The average amount of water in an adult male is 45 l. Water is present in different compartments in the body. Around 30 l of water will be found inside the cells of the body and the remaining 15 l will be found outside the cells. The main purpose of water in the body is to help in the transport of waste and the production of digestive and lubricating fluids, maintaining hydration of body tissues and temperature control through sweating. To maintain good hydration, the body requires between 2 and 3 l of water daily and must be in balance with any fluid loss in the form of urine and faeces.

Vitamins
Vitamins are required for the body to help maintain metabolism. The body only requires trace amounts of vitamins, which are

Table 10.1 Different types of vitamins.

Water-soluble vitamins	Fat-soluble vitamins
Vitamin B_1	Vitamin A
Vitamin B_2	Vitamin D
Vitamin B_6	Vitamin E
Vitamin B_{12}	Vitamin K
Vitamin C	

divided into water-soluble and fat-soluble vitamins. See Table 10.1 for different types of vitamins.

Functions of water-soluble vitamins

Vitamin B_1 is also known as thiamine. It helps with the absorption of carbohydrates. Vitamin B_2 is also known as riboflavin and is needed to maintain the normal function of cell enzymes. Vitamin B_6 helps in the absorption of proteins. Intrinsic factor is produced by the stomach and aids in the absorption of vitamin B_{12}. Vitamin B_{12} is essential in the development of red blood cells in the bone marrow and the nervous system.

Functions of fat-soluble vitamins

Vitamin A is found in carrots and tomatoes and is required for the normal functioning of the retina and to fight infections. Vitamin D is found in dairy products and can be absorbed through the uncovered skin via sunshine rays. Vitamin D works together with calcium to maintain bones. Vitamin E is found in egg yolks and milk and is required in the muscles, nerves and development of the reproductory organs. Vitamin K is found in green vegetables and liver. It is needed to produce blood clotting factors in the liver.

Minerals

Minerals are known as *salts* or *electrolytes*. Minerals are essential for normal metabolism and have the ability to conduct electrical charges down nerves and muscles. Sodium and potassium are important electrolytes within the body. They are important for the maintenance of fluid balance and the conduction of electrical impulses within the nervous system. Calcium is also required for the proper functioning of nerves and muscles. Iron is needed to form haemoglobin in red blood cells. Iodine is needed to help in the formation of thyroxine by the thyroid gland.

WHAT IS METABOLISM?

Metabolism refers to the chemical changes that occur within the body to convert food into fuel. This fuel is then used by the body to create energy to move, talk, walk, think, sleep, heal and repair itself. Another way of thinking about metabolism is to think of the body as a big chemical factory. Raw materials of food are passed through many different chemical processes (via the GI tract) before they are in the right chemical form to be utilised by the body. The body's cells then use glucose and oxygen to create energy (fuel). Food is a vital fuel source used by the body, which will provide energy to feed cells, build and repair tissues, as well as regulate metabolism.

What happens to metabolism in illness?

When a person becomes sick, the metabolic rate increases. Think of a time when you or a close friend has been unwell with a sore throat, flu or chickenpox. The body recognises that there is an infection and tries to fight it off by increasing the metabolic rate. This increases the demand for fuel by using up any glucose (the body's fuel) already in the blood stream and then tapping into the glycogen stores it has stored already in the liver. Once these are used up, the body will then turn to any fat stores available in the body and convert that into glucose. When the fat stores are all empty, the body will use up its muscle stores. Once all stores of carbohydrates, fats and proteins are used up, the body will try to maintain metabolism using up its own cells and tissues. If only glucose is used to create fuel for the body, then *anaerobic metabolism* occurs. Anaerobic metabolism produces a waste called *lactic acid*.

An example of anaerobic metabolism is when you run fast and get a painful stitch in the side because there is not enough oxygen available to combine with the glucose to create energy to maintain the running pace. There is a short supply of oxygen, which affects the chemical process and so you slow down your running pace to breathe quicker to get more oxygen in. To remain in a constant anaerobic metabolic state is bad for the body and eventually death will occur.

DEFINITION OF MALNUTRITION

Weller (2005, p. 242) defines malnutrition as 'The condition in which nutrition is defective in quantity or quality'. NICE (2006, p. 21) defined malnutrition as, 'A state of nutrition in which a deficiency of energy, protein and/or other nutrients causes measurable adverse effects on tissue/body form, composition, function or clinical outcome'. NICE (2006, p. 151) goes on to further qualify this definition by outlining guidelines for identifying people at risk of malnutrition. These are listed below:

- A BMI less than $18.5 \, kg/m^2$.
- Unintentional loss of greater than 10% body weight within the previous 3–6 months.
- The patient has eaten little or nothing for more than 5 days and/or is likely to eat little or nothing for the next 5 days or longer.
- The patient has poor absorptive capacity, is catabolic and/or has high nutrient losses and/or has increased nutritional needs.

THE EFFECTS OF POOR NUTRITION ON HEALTH AND THE RECOVERY OF PATIENTS

A balanced diet, fluids and exercise are an important way to prevent ill health and maintain good health. There are many factors that influence why patients do not always have a balanced diet (see Table 10.2).

Within the United Kingdom, it is estimated that there are 2 million adults who are malnourished. It has been suggested that between 15 and 40% of acute admissions to hospital already have a pre-existing problem with malnutrition. Dehydration is a common problem as well.

If people do not have a balanced diet, then this can delay recovery in someone when ill. Lack of a balanced diet will impact on the body's immune system and people can become vulnerable to infection. The skin can begin to easily break down and this can put patients at risk of pressure sores. The metabolic rate is increased in illness, which leads to a rapid weight loss, as the body

Table 10.2 Influences on poor nutrition.

Poverty – lack of money for food. Fresh food is expensive
Lifestyle – smoking, drinking and lack of exercise
Education – poor nutrients in school dinners or
sandwiches. Unhealthy food choices
Personal choice
Family influences – parents, peers what they do
Body image – perception of self, over- or undereating
Underlying illness – acute or chronic diseases

uses up all its energy stores. When the glucose stores of the body are empty, this has the knock-on effect of making a person feel dizzy and lethargic. They may find it difficult to find the energy to do anything from getting out of bed, walking around, lifting or carrying things. This can lead to reduced motivation and some people can become depressed and withdrawn and demonstrate personality changes.

So, how can we improve the nutritional status of patients? Well, it must first of all start with a nutritional assessment.

The role of nutritional screening and assessment tools

In 2006, the National Institute for Clinical Excellence (NICE) outlined some recommendations for healthcare workers to use when dealing with nutritional problems of patients. They are called *Nutrition support in adults: oral nutrition support, enteral tube feeding and parenteral nutrition*, Clinical Guideline 32.

Within the NICE (2006, p. 38) document, there is emphasis that 'People with malnutrition should have the opportunity to make informed decisions about their care and treatment, in partnership with their healthcare professionals'. Patients should be actively involved in the planning and implementation of their nutritional care. In 2007, the DH published *Improving Nutritional Care*, which is a document that outlines their action plan to tackle nutritional problems. The document (2007, p. 8) outlines '10 Key characteristics for good nutritional care in hospitals'. The 10 key characteristics are outlined in Box 10.1. The author suggests that these 10 characteristics could be applied to nursing and residential care homes within the community setting as well as within the private sector.

Box 10.1 Ten key characteristics of good nutritional care in hospitals

1. All patients are screened on admission to identify those who are malnourished or at risk of becoming malnourished. All patients are re-screened weekly.
2. All patients have a care plan, which identifies their nutritional care needs and how they are to be met.
3. The hospital includes specific guidance on food services and nutritional care in its clinical governance arrangements.
4. Patients are involved in the planning and monitoring arrangements for food service provision.
5. The ward implements protected mealtimes to provide an environment conducive to patients enjoying and being able to eat their food.
6. All staff have the appropriate skills and competencies needed to ensure that patient's nutritional needs are met. All staff receive regular training on nutritional care and management.
7. Hospital facilities are designed to be flexible and patient centred with the aim of providing and delivering an excellent experience of food service and nutritional care 24 hours a day, every day.
8. The hospital has a policy for food service and nutritional care that is patient centred and its performance managed in line with home country governance frameworks.
9. Food service and nutritional care are delivered to the patient safely.
10. The hospital supports a multidisciplinary approach to nutritional care and values the contribution of all staff groups working in partnership with patients and users.

Practice point 10.1

Using the 10 key characteristics of good nutritional care as your guide, find out if your workplace (hospital, nursing home or residential home) has mechanisms in place to achieve all of the 10 key areas. If not, think about ways in which this can be changed and improved and talk to your senior nurse or manager about it.

Nutritional screening should commence on admission whether in hospital or nursing home. During the admission process, it is important to gather as much information from the patients about their lifestyle and eating habits. You may approach the person who is admitting the patient and glean information about their nutritional status using the look, listen and feel approach.

Look

Look at the patient and notice whether they look a healthy size or whether they are under- or overweight. You may notice that their clothes are fitting well or that they are too big for them. Look at their skin and nails. Does the skin look healthy and hydrated? Does the skin look sunburnt, suntanned or pale? Is the skin intact or is there a broken area of the skin or long-standing leg ulcers? What do the hands and nails look like? Are the hands healthy, or do the fingers have swollen joints due to arthritis? Are the fingers discoloured from nicotine stains? If the patient is undressed or you are washing the patient, look at the state of the skin all over the body and also at the state of the feet and toenails. Does the patient walk well or require assistance? Poor mobility and dexterity may impact on the ability to exercise or walk to the kitchen or carry a cup of tea or a plate of food.

Listen

Listen to the patients when they describe their medical and lifestyle history. You can gather so much information from them about how much they eat, drink and exercise. Listen carefully when the patients talk about their bowel habits. For example, a constipated patient may not be drinking enough fluid or may be lacking in enough fibre in the diet. A patient with diarrhoea may have an infection, but diarrhoea causes fluid and electrolyte losses and so the patient may need to increase the fluid intake to compensate for the loss. It may be necessary to commence the patient on a Bristol Stool Chart to record and monitor the consistency and frequency of stools.

They may tell you what they weigh. People often under- or overestimate what their weight is or never weigh themselves at all. At some point in the assessment and nutritional screening process, the patients will need to be weighed. The patients may be able to tell you how much they weigh, but it is important to get an objective assessment by weighing as well as finding out the height of the patients. This will allow you to calculate the body mass index (BMI).

Feel

During the nutritional screening process, it is useful to touch and feel the skin of the patient. The skin may be dry and flake when you touch it, which may be a sign of dry and dehydrated skin. Sometimes, when you touch the skin you may leave imprints of your fingers. This may be due to oedema and this may be a sign of illness and will therefore put your patient at a high risk of malnutrition.

Having gathered information from talking and listening to your patient, you must then write this information in the patient's care plan and record in the nutritional screening tool. Many hospitals and health centres have adopted or adapted the Malnutrition Universal Screening Tool (MUST) from the British Association for Parenteral and Enteral Nutrition (BAPEN, 2003) (Fig. 10.2).

Body mass index

You need to know your weight in kilograms and your height in metres. The formula for calculating your BMI is *by dividing the weight in kilograms by the height in metres squared* (NICE, 2006). To get the height in metres squared, multiply the number by itself.

BMI less than 19 – underweight.
BMI between 19 and 25 – in normal weight range
BMI more than 25–30 – overweight
BMI more than 30 – obese

When using BMI you should take into account the body shape and muscle mass. For example, an Olympic athlete may have a BMI greater than 25 because of their muscle bulk, as muscle weighs more than fat, but we all know that they are super fit and healthy.

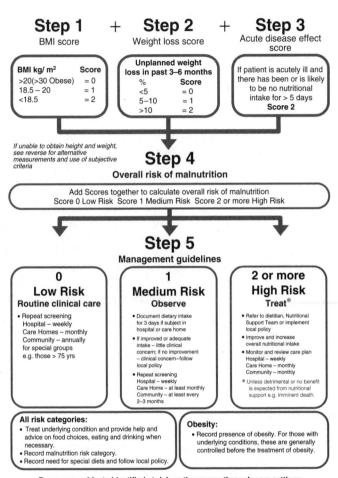

Step 1 + **Step 2** + **Step 3**
BMI score   Weight loss score   Acute disease effect
                                                score

BMI kg/m²	Score
>20(>30 Obese)	= 0
18.5 – 20	= 1
<18.5	= 2

Unplanned weight loss in past 3–6 months	
%	Score
<5	= 0
5–10	= 1
>10	= 2

If patient is acutely ill and there has been or is likely to be no nutritional intake for > 5 days
Score 2

If unable to obtain height and weight, see reverse for alternative measurements and use of subjective criteria

Step 4
Overall risk of malnutrition

Add Scores together to calculate overall risk of malnutrition
Score 0 Low Risk Score 1 Medium Risk Score 2 or more High Risk

Step 5
Management guidelines

0
Low Risk
Routine clinical care
- Repeat screening
  Hospital – weekly
  Care Homes – monthly
  Community – annually
  for special groups
  e.g. those > 75 yrs

1
Medium Risk
Observe
- Document dietary intake for 3 days if subject in hospital or care home
- If improved or adequate intake – little clinical concern; if no improvement – clinical concern–follow local policy
- Repeat screening
  Hospital – weekly
  Care Home – at least monthly
  Community – at least every 2–3 months

2 or more
High Risk
Treat*
- Refer to dietitian, Nutritional Support Team or implement local policy
- Improve and increase overall nutritional intake
- Monitor and review care plan
  Hospital – weekly
  Care Home – monthly
  Community – monthly
* Unless detrimental or no benefit is expected from nutritional support e.g. imminent death.

All risk categories:
- Treat underlying condition and provide help and advice on food choices, eating and drinking when necessary.
- Record malnutrition risk category.
- Record need for special diets and follow local policy.

Obesity:
- Record presence of obesity. For those with underlying conditions, these are generally controlled before the treatment of obesity.

Re-assess subjects identified at risk as they move through care settings

See The 'MUST' Explanatory Booklet for further details and The 'MUST' Reportfor supporting evidence.

Fig. 10.2 The Malnutrition Universal Screening Tool (MUST tool). Reproduced with permission from BAPEN.

Another way to know if your health is at risk is by measuring your waist size. Your *health is at risk* if you waist is

(a) 40 inch plus for a Caucasian male;
(b) 38 inch plus for an Asian male;
(c) 35 inch plus for a Caucasian female;
(d) 32 inch plus for an Asian female.

The NICE (2006) guidelines define a person as malnourished if they have a BMI of less than $18.5 \, kg/m^2$; unintentional weight loss greater than 10% within the last 3–6 months or a BMI of less than $20 \, kg/m^2$ with unintentional weight loss greater than 5% within the last 3–6 months.

Patients may be at risk of malnutrition if they have eaten little or nothing for more than 5 days and are likely to eat little or nothing for the next 5 days or longer. Another group of people who may be at risk of malnutrition are those who have a poor absorption capacity, high nutrient losses (such as vomiting or diarrhoea) and increased nutritional needs from causes such as catabolism (NICE, 2006). Using the MUST tool or an adapted version enables healthcare staff to obtain a baseline assessment of the patient's current nutritional condition and will highlight the need for seeking further advice and management from either a dietician or other experts such as the speech and language therapist. Once the assessment is completed, a nutritional management plan can be implemented. All patients require nutritional intake via the oral, enteral or parenteral route.

ORAL NUTRITION

If there is no clinical reason why a person cannot eat or drink, then ultimately the oral route for nutritional intake is the best route. This is because it is the most natural way in which food is broken down into fuel, and eating things via the oral route will stimulate the whole of the digestive system to work and prevent further complications. People need to have the ability to chew and swallow to use this route and they can also make healthy choices when maintaining a balanced diet of carbohydrates, fats, proteins, vitamins and minerals. Therefore, staff should promote patients to attend to any oral hygiene care such as brushing of teeth or cleaning dentures. If any swallowing difficulties are observed, then it may be useful to refer the patient to the speech and language therapist. If patients have problems with cutting up food or using cutlery because of pain or damaged hands and fingers, it may be useful to refer the patient to the occupational therapy staff who can assist in obtaining adapted cutlery, plates and cups.

ENTERAL ROUTE

If a patient is unable to maintain the nutritional intake with the oral route or cannot eat or drink orally for whatever reason, then nutrients must be administered using the enteral route. The dietician will prescribe the type of feed required. This means that nutrients are delivered directly into the stomach, duodenum or jejunum using a feeding tube that has been inserted by either a doctor or a trained nurse. The enteral route can only be used if the digestive system is intact and able to function normally.

The most common method of delivering the nutrients is via a nasogastric (NG) tube. The NG tube is usually passed through the nose down the oesophagus and into the stomach. It can be an uncomfortable procedure for patients and they require lots of support and reassurance to tolerate it. Food is delivered through sterile packages with liquids that are made up of the right amount of nutrients.

The enteral route is useful for post-operative patients with limited oral intake. There is research that suggests that early enteral feeding after planned surgery or cancer surgery will reduce post-operative complications and reduce the patient's stay in hospital (Bozzetti et al., 2001; Stroud et al., 2003). Should there be long-term need for using the enteral route, then enteral feeding can be used through the percutaneous endoscopic gastrotomy (PEG) route or the percutaneous endoscopic jejunostomy (PEJ) route.

PEG or PEJ feeding is commonly found within community settings for people with long-term nutritional problems. The key reason for this is dysphagia, following a stroke or in people with multiple sclerosis (MS) or motor neuron disease (MND).

To prevent the tubes from blockage, it is essential that they are flushed with sterile water prior to commencing the feed and whenever any medications are administered via this route (Dougherty and Lister, 2008).

Some side effects experienced using the enteral feeding route include bloating and cramps in the abdomen, nausea, diarrhoea and constipation. This happens because the normal physiological mechanisms (chewing and release of digestive enzymes) are bypassed. Seek the advice of the dietician before stopping the feeding regime, as there may be an alternative feed preparation that could be used or the doctor can prescribe some medicines to promote gut motility.

Good hygiene and infection control are important to prevent any spread of infection via the enteral route. This includes good hand-washing practice, use of gloves to prepare the feed and changing of the enteral feeding line and feed bag every 24 hours.

Parenteral route

Patients who cannot use the oral or enteral route to obtain their nutritional requirements will require total parenteral nutrition (TPN).

NICE (2006) recommends that the parenteral feeding route should be used in all patients who are clinically assessed to be malnourished or at risk of malnutrition. It should also be used in people who have a non-functioning or compromised digestive tract. Parenteral feeding is administered directly into the vein via an intravenous drip. It may be used as a supplement to oral or enteral feeding or as the only source of TPN and can be found in the acute hospital or community settings.

TPN can be administered through a large central vein or a peripheral vein. Both central and peripheral veins must be cannulated using strict aseptic technique either by the specialist nurse in nutrition or a doctor trained in these skills. The TPN drip should be dedicated only to the administration of the feed and never used for taking blood samples or administration of intravenous medications. Specially prepared bags of TPN are made up by the pharmacists, which are between 1 and 2.5 l. They are run via an infusion pump over a varied time frame (between 18- and 24-hour periods), and strict hand hygiene must be maintained when handling the intravenous drip to prevent the risk of infection as discussed in the Chapter 2.

THE ROLE OF THE NURSE IN MONITORING AND REPORTING THE NUTRITIONAL INTAKE OF PATIENTS

Nursing staff are often the people who are the first line of contact with the patient and so are ideally placed to monitor and report any problems to the dietician or the doctor.

Nursing staff may admit the patients and will be able to discuss with the patients their weight, their dietary habits and whether there is a preexisting problem with nutrition. The stress of admission to hospital or illness will influence patients about whether or not they want to eat or drink. It has been reported that some patients feel lonely and isolated on entering the ward area and this may result in a refusal to eat (Lloyd and Moody, 1999). Noisy ward areas and clinical activity can inhibit nutritional intake.

There are several ways to promote compliance with a balanced nutritional intake. These include creating a dining experience for a patient, which takes into account the way food is prepared and presented as well as the place where food is eaten. For example, some places have dedicated dining rooms that encourage the patient to interact with other patients away from the bedside. Sometimes, building in a routine for a patient helps in planning activities and mealtimes because eating should be a social and enjoyable experience and has prompted the Department of Health (2007) to recommend 'protected mealtimes'.

At mealtimes, patients should be protected from clinical activity such as ward rounds, medicines rounds, bed baths and diagnostic tests. A study by Eastwood (1997) found that between 11 and 27% of patients missed meals. The reason for this includes clinical investigations, illness or the poor quality of the food. Most recently, Welsh (2007) videotaped mealtimes and found that the staff did not recognise or realise how their clinical activities impacted on the patients. Welsh (2007) observed ritualised practices where the staff started distributing the meals at the same place each day and therefore patients receiving their food at the end of the meal round were served lukewarm or even cold food. Many meals were wrapped in cellophane wrappers and the staff did not always remove these for patients who needed assistance. Food was placed out of the reach of the patients. Some patients did complain and one patient described the meal as 'a kid's portion' (Welsh, 2007, p. 130). This action learning study did bring about change in staff behaviour and the study resulted in change of the clinical routine. This was also videotaped and this showed increased interaction between staff and patients, assistance to patients and patients' choices and patients getting second helping if they wanted.

Protected mealtimes ensure that nurses focus on promoting good nutritional intake. It is an ideal time to observe exactly what a patient is eating and even an opportunity to provide some healthy eating information to aid the patients in their recovery. The protected mealtime concept also allows the nurse to identify the patients with special needs (O'Regan, 2009). There should be food provision for patients in hospital 24 hours a day (The Council of Europe Committee of Ministers, 2003), and therefore, this may mean providing additional meals or snack boxes. Patients should be able to make informed choices about their nutritional needs and should be able to access drinks and snacks at any time.

Some patients require support to eat; they may require their food to be cut up or assistance to eat because they have problems with their arms and hands. Some hospitals have implemented the coloured tray scheme as a mechanism to aid staff in identifying the patients who require assistance at mealtimes. Any food that is taken should be monitored, as this will guide the dietician and nursing staff about the amount of calories that have been eaten to create fuel and energy for the body. Food diaries are a good way to record how much diet is taken as well as a method of assessing patient's food choices. It is important that fluid intake is also recorded, as hydration is an essential component of nutrition. Any concerns observed by the junior nurse or healthcare assistant should be reported to the nurse in charge.

CONCLUSION

This chapter has discussed the role and importance of nutrition within clinical observations to aid in the health and recovery of patients in the healthcare setting. Patients who are malnourished will be lethargic and at higher risk of clinical deterioration. O'Regan (2009, p. 41) suggests that 'Feeding and providing nutrition is not a medical treatment, but a basic human need'. The nursing team are an essential part of the multidisciplinary approach in the assessment, monitoring and management of nutritional needs of patients.

REFERENCES

Bozzetti F, Braga M, Gianotti L, Gavazzi C, and Mariani L (2001). Postoperative enteral versus parenteral nutrition in malnourished patients with gastrointestinal cancer. A randomised multicentre trial. *Lancet* **358**(9292), 1487–1492.

British Association for Parenteral and Enteral Nutrition (BAPEN) (2003). *The 'MUST' Explanatory Booklet. A Guide to the 'Malnutrition Universal Screening Tool' (MUST) for Adults.* BAPEN Website www.bapen.org.uk.

British Association for Parenteral and Enteral Nutrition (BAPEN) (2006). *The 'MUST' Explanatory Booklet. A Guide to the 'Malnutrition Universal Screening Tool' (MUST) for Adults.* BAPEN Website www.bapen.org.uk.

Council of Europe. Committee of Ministers (2003). Resolution ResAP(2003)3 on food and nutritional care in hospital. https://wcd.coe.int/wcd.

Department of Health (2007). *Improving Nutritional Care. A Joint Action Plan from the Department of Health and Nutrition Summit stakeholders.* London, Department of Health.

Dougherty L and Lister S (2008). *The Royal Marsden Hospital Manual of Clinical Nursing Procedures.* 7th edn. Oxford, Wiley-Blackwell.

Eastwood M (1997). Hospital food. *New England Journal of Medicine* **336**(17), 1261–1262.

Grodner M, Long S and deYoung S (2004). *Foundations and clinical applications of nutrition. A Nursing Approach.* St Louis, Mosby, Inc.

Lloyd N and Moody M (1999). Nutrition: a fundamental human need. *Nursing and Residential Care* **1**(3), 145.

National Institute for Clinical Excellence (2006). *Nutrition Support in Adults, Oral Nutrition Support, Enteral Tube Feeding and Parenteral Nutrition.* Clinical Guideline32. London, NICE. www.nice.org.

O'Regan P (2009). Nutrition for patients in hospital. *Nursing Standard* **23**(23), 35–41.

Smith G and Watson R (2006). *Gastrointestinal Nursing.* Oxford, Blackwell Publishing Ltd.

Stroud M, Duncan H, and Nightingale J (2003). Guidelines for enteral feeding in adult patients. *Gut* **52**(VII) 1.

Waugh A and Grant A (2001). *Ross and Wilson Anatomy and Physiology in Health and Illness.* 9th edn. London, Churchill Livingstone.

Weller BF (2005). *Baillere's Nurses' Dictionary for Nurses and Health Care Workers.* 24th edn. London, Elsevier.

Welsh R (2007). Mealtimes with the elderly: results of videotaped research. *British Journal of Healthcare Assistants* **1**(3), 129–132.

FURTHER READING

Department of Health (2001). *Food and Nutrition. The Essence of Care. Patient Focused Benchmarking for Health Care Practitioners.* 76–97. www.dh.gov.uk.

Medicines and Healthcare Products Regulatory Agency (2004). *Enteral Feeding Tubes (Nasogastric).* MDA bulletin 2004/026. www.mhra.gov.uk.

Methany N (2002). Risk factors for aspiration. *Journal of Parenteral and Enteral Nutrition* **26**(6), S26–S31.

Nath S, Hack SL, Roberts PH, and Clutton-Brock TH (2002). Enteral and parenteral nutrition. In: *Fundamental Principles and Practice of Anaesthesia.* 1st edn. London, Martin Dunitz Ltd.

National Collaborating Centre for Acute Care (2006). *Nutrition Support in Adults. Oral Nutrition Support, Enteral Tube Feeding and Parenteral Nutrition. Methods, Evidence and Guidance.* The National Collaborating Centre for Acute Care at the Royal College of Surgeons of England. www.nice.org.uk.

National Nursing, Midwifery and Health Visiting Advisory Committee (2002). *Promoting Nutrition for Older Adult in Patients in NHS Hospitals in Scotland.* Scottish Executive Health Department, 1–38. www.scotland.gov.uk/library.

Blood Glucose Monitoring

11

INTRODUCTION

Blood glucose monitoring is an important part of the patient's vital signs and is central to the assessment process. Glucose is required by the body to maintain the body's metabolism, and any deviation from the normal range may result in an altered level of consciousness in the patient. Obtaining a sample of blood from the patient is the first step towards measuring the glucose levels within the body.

LEARNING OUTCOMES

By the end of this chapter, you will be able to discuss the following:

❑ The anatomy and physiology related to blood glucose
❑ Stress response
❑ Abnormal/normal blood glucose readings
❑ Diabetes
❑ How to perform equipments checks/quality control test
❑ How to obtain a capillary blood sample
❑ Cleaning and storage of the glucose monitor
❑ Documentation
❑ Policies and guidelines

ANATOMY AND PHYSIOLOGY

The two major glands within our body that are involved in maintaining blood glucose levels are the liver and the pancreas. The

Vital Signs for Nurses: An Introduction to Clinical Observations, First Edition.
Joyce Smith and Rachel Roberts.
© 2011 Joyce Smith and Rachel Roberts. Published 2011 by Blackwell Publishing Ltd.

liver is the largest gland in the body and the portal vein enters the liver, carrying blood from the stomach and pancreas. The *pancreas* is a pale grey gland that is about 12–15 cm long and lies behind the stomach (Waugh and Grant, 2006). Within the gland are specialised cells that are called the Islets of Langerhans that produce the hormones insulin and glucagon. The beta cells secrete insulin to promote carbohydrate metabolism and the alpha cells secrete glucagon that stimulates *glycogenolysis* in the liver (Watkins et al., 2003). Both hormones are stimulated by fluctuating blood glucose levels that flow directly into the blood stream. These two hormones work together to regulate blood glucose levels, ensuring that they are maintained within the normal range of 4–7 mmol/l (Ferguson, 2005). For our brain to function effectively, it needs both oxygen and glucose. Glucose is the only fuel that the brain cells use; however, the brain does not have the ability to store glucose; therefore, it needs a constant supply of glucose provided by the blood to function properly (Tortora and Nielsen, 2009).

WHAT IS BLOOD GLUCOSE?

Metabolism refers to the chemical changes that occur within the body to convert food into fuel and to create energy. Food is a vital fuel used by the body that provides energy to feed cells, build and repair tissues as well as regulate metabolism. Our body obtains glucose (sugar) from the breakdown of carbohydrates within the gut. Once the glucose has been absorbed from the gut into the blood stream, excess glucose travels to the liver and is converted and stored as glycogen. However, if the blood sugar level in our body drops (*hypoglycaemia*), the glycogen that is stored in the liver can be converted back to glucose (glycogenolysis) and released into the bloodstream to restore blood sugar levels to the normal range.

A rise of blood glucose stimulates the pancreas to release the hormone insulin, which allows glucose to enter cells. Insulin is like a key that unlocks the 'door' to the cells, to allow the glucose to enter. Once inside the cells the glucose is used to create energy; this is part of the Krebs cycle. Again, as previously discussed, any excessive amount of glucose maybe sent to the liver for storage in the form of glycogen (Higgins, 2008). The body also gets rid of excessive glucose by storing it as fat or by excreting it through the kidneys in the form of urine. A drop in glucose alerts the pancreas to produce the hormone glucagon that stimulates the liver to release the glycogen back into the blood stream. If no carbohydrate source is found by the body, then it will use the fat stores. Other factors such as psychological or physiological stressors may affect metabolism, creating a metabolic imbalance that influences the body's hormone levels. The body has a natural metabolic response to stressors and releases hormones that result in the sympathetic nervous system creating a fight or flight reaction to help the body cope with stressful situations. The hormones adrenaline and noradrenaline, collectively known as *catecholamines*, are released into the blood stream during the fight or flight reaction. The adrenal cortex produces glucocorticoids (cortisol) that promote cell metabolism and help the body to cope with prolonged or continuing stressors. The hormone levels rise in response to the stressors and unless the stressor is relieved, the body cannot continue to compensate.

WHAT IS THE STRESS RESPONSE?

Stress is a normal response to trauma, illness or any life event. It is normally a mechanism for adapting to problems or changed circumstances. Anxiety and associated stress can have unfortunate short- or long-term effects that can be mild and reversible but may become chronic. This is because of the physiological response to stress called the *general adaptation syndrome*, first described by Hans Selyé (1956), which occurs in three stages.

Stage One: Alarm stage – also known as 'fight or flight' (Marieb, 2009). This is a quickly occurring nervous (sympathetic autonomic nervous system (ANS)) system response that results in a raised metabolism, raised blood sugar, increased alertness and increased muscle tone.

Stage two: Resistance (or adaptation) – this is a slower and more sustainable endocrine system response. The metabolism is raised and therefore blood sugar levels are raised and there is an increase in cortisone level.

Stage three: Exhaustion – when the body has run out of resources to sustain the responses, a person can become glucose intolerant and physically exhausted and tissue deterioration sets in (Braun and Anderson, 2007).

WHY DO WE NEED TO MONITOR OUR BLOOD GLUCOSE?

The brain needs a constant supply of glucose to maintain metabolic activity and cellular function; therefore, the brain is sensitive to any changes in the blood glucose level. A patient who is severely stressed by an acute illness or who has sustained a head injury will potentially have an altered metabolic response. The stress response stimulates glycogen and fat to break down, causing the blood glucose levels to rise. Therefore, when a patient is acutely ill, more glucose is released into the blood and insulin is prevented from working properly. As there is not enough insulin to regulate the glucose, the levels remain high.

In a patient who has no known neurological injury but has an altered level of consciousness, there is a metabolic imbalance caused by alterations in the blood sugar levels (McLeod, 2006). The patient may also display signs of confusion and agitation; therefore, obtaining a blood sample and checking the glucose levels will provide valuable information in identifying whether the patient is hypo- or hyperglycaemic. Tortora and Nielsen (2009) state that the brain requires approximately 20% of glucose at rest, and a reduced blood supply to the brain may result in an altered level of consciousness. In addition, low levels of glucose within the blood will have the same effect on the patient's level of consciousness. One possible consequence of continuous ongoing stress is that the patient may develop diabetes (insulin resistant).

DIABETES

In the hospital, community or private healthcare setting, you may care for patients who have been diagnosed as diabetics. Often patients may require more frequent blood sugar monitoring. Reasons for this include illness, lifestyle or insufficient knowledge on how to manage their blood sugar levels. There are an estimated 2.35 million people with diabetes in England and this is expected to increase to more than 2.5 million by 2010 (DH, 2008). Diabetes is recognised as a chronic long-term condition and is defined as 'health problems that require ongoing management over a period of years or decades' (World Health Organisation (WHO), 2005, p. 13). The word diabetes is derived from Greek and means 'a syphoning of water through the body' ('because the fluid does not remain in the body but uses the body as a channel whereby to leave it') (Williams and Pickup, 2004, p. 6). The rising number of people with diabetes has also been linked to obesity; in England, there are already over 1 million obese children under the age of 16, thereby increasing the potential number of people who will be diagnosed with diabetes (British Medical Association (BMA), 2007). The World Health Organisation (WHO) has classified diabetes mellitus into two major types according to whether insulin therapy is essential or not. Type 1 diabetes is insulin dependent whereas type 2 is non-insulin dependent; however, it is also possible that patients who are diagnosed with type 2 may also need insulin (WHO, 2005).

Patients cared for in the hospital, community or private health sector may have type 1 or type 2 diabetes mellitus. Diabetes mellitus is a common term associated with diabetics; the term mellitus means 'sweet as honey' (Tortora and Nielsen, 2009). Diabetes mellitus is a condition in which the concentration of blood glucose is raised. It is caused because the body does not produce the hormone insulin or because of insufficient levels of insulin or when the insulin produced within the body does not function properly (insulin resistance). In your practice area, you will meet patients who are diabetics or newly diagnosed diabetics who need to monitor their blood glucose levels at regular intervals. Diabetic patients control their blood sugar levels by either diet or exercise or a combination of diet and insulin injection or diet with oral medication. If the pancreas does not produce enough insulin, the level of glucose in the body rises. In a healthy person, the blood glucose level is between 4 and 7 mmol (Cowan, 1997). Monitoring the patient's blood glucose will provide you with important information and an indication of when the blood glucose levels are not within the normal range.

Type 1 diabetes mellitus

Type 1 diabetes is a result of insulin deficiency as the body is unable to produce the hormone insulin and is usually diagnosed in childhood or in young adults. The patient requires insulin that is administered either by a pen injection device or a needle into the subcutaneous tissue. Patients who are established diabetics will monitor their capillary blood glucose as and when it is required. Insulin pens are a popular choice for injections as the insulin is contained in the barrel of the pen and the pens have a fine needle. In certain circumstances continuous subcutaneous insulin infusion (CSII or 'Insulin Pump') therapy is considered as a treatment option for adults with type 1 diabetes mellitus if they are unable to control their blood glucose levels. However, the National Institute for Clinical Excellence (2008) states that CSII OR 'Insulin Pump' therapy should only be started by a trained specialist team (NICE, 2008). The signs and symptoms associated with type 1 diabetes can develop quickly and a consistent high blood glucose level may result in diabetic ketoacidosis (DKA). This may happen when the patient becomes acutely ill because there is insufficient glucose entering the cells to meet the body's energy requirements. The body begins to use stores of fat as an alternative source of energy; this then produces an acidic by-product known as *ketones* (Dunning, 2003). When ketones are present and blood glucose levels are rising, patients may become increasingly thirsty. Glucose is excreted by the kidneys, and this results in increased urine production as the body tries to flush the ketones out. It may be possible to smell ketones on the patients' breath, as it is often described as smelling like pear drops or nail varnish. A simple reagent test will confirm whether ketones are present in the urine. If untreated, the level of ketones will continue to rise and, combined with high blood glucose levels, coma will develop, which potentially can be fatal. The patient will need emergency treatment of insulin and fluids to address the uncontrolled blood glucose levels. All patients who have diabetes and require insulin therapy may potentially develop DKA.

DKA is a medical emergency and the signs and symptoms that may be observed in type 1 or type 2 diabetics include deep and rapid respirations called *Kussmaul's respiration* (as previously discussed, the respiratory rate is the most sensitive indicator that the patient may be developing a potential problem) and become hypotensive. The odour of pear drops or acetone may be present on the patient's breath and protein may also be present in the urine sample (Watkins et al., 2003). High glucose readings in capillary blood will be observed and other signs and symptoms may also include

- exceptional thirst,
- dry mouth,
- frequent urination,

- loss of weight,
- weakness or fatigue,
- blurred vision.

There is no clear cause of type 1 diabetes, although genetic factors and environmental influences have been identified and linked to type 1 diabetes and treatment requires lifelong supplemental insulin (NICE, 2004a).

Type 2 diabetes mellitus

The majority of people who are diagnosed with type 2 diabetes are in the age group of over 40 – the elderly; type 2 diabetes is the most common form of diabetes (Williams and Pickup, 2004). In type 2 diabetes, patients have a deficiency of insulin and, more commonly, a resistance (hyperglycaemia – when the pancreas insulin reserve is unable to meet the body's demands) for insulin; although the body can still produce insulin, it fails to produce sufficient levels (Watkins et al., 2003). It is suggested that obesity and genetics may be a factor in developing type 2 diabetes; equally, the growing trend of obesity in young children has resulted in children now being diagnosed with type 2 diabetes (NICE, 2004b; BMA, 2007). Type 2 diabetes may be controlled by a combination of diet and exercise or diet, exercise and oral tablets. In your practice area, patients may be prescribed a tablet called *metformin* that helps to control their blood glucose levels. When metformin (or other oral hypoglycaemic drugs) can no longer control the blood glucose level, patients may also require insulin.

The signs and symptoms for type 2 diabetes are listed below:

- Blurred vision
- Cuts or sores that take a long time to heal
- Itching skin or yeast infections
- Excessive thirst
- Dry mouth
- Frequent urination
- Leg pain

The risk factors associated with type 2 diabetes include age, family history, obesity, lack of physical activity and diet. Diet is an important part of the management of all patients who are diagnosed as either type 1 or type 2 diabetics, as they need to control their blood glucose levels. Therefore, educating patients on their diet or referral to a dietician is an essential part of the care management in helping patients to control their blood sugar levels (NICE, 2004b).

Patients who are either type 1 or type 2 diabetics may also develop hypoglycaemia or hyperglycaemia. *Hypoglycaemia* (Hypo = low, glyce = glucose and emia = blood) occurs when the blood glucose level is very low and often has a rapid onset. Signs that you may observe in your patients are sweating, trembling, headache and confusion. A sugary drink may be all that is needed; in your practice area, you may have a sugar box (Fig. 11.1). The brain depends on glucose as its fuel source and if the brain does not receive enough glucose, the patient will become drowsy and confused (Dunning, 2003). Immediate treatment is needed or the patient may become unconscious. It is important that you inform a senior member of the healthcare team because if the blood glucose is found to be below 3 mmol/l, intravenous dextrose should be

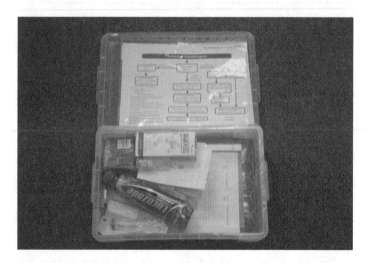

Fig. 11.1 Hypoglycaemia box (photograph).

administered and the blood glucose levels checked again after 15 minutes (Resuscitation Council UK (RSC), 2006).

Practice point 11.1

Mrs Brown is a 48-year-old who has been admitted with a 2-day history of nausea and vomiting. She has recently been diagnosed with type 2 diabetes. On admission, you take her clinical observations and notice that she is triggering a score on the Early Warning Scoring (EWS) of 5. Her respiratory rate is 30, heart rate is 120, and blood pressure is 170/80; she is alert but slightly confused and sweating. When you check her blood glucose, it is 2.8 mmol.

Q1. What do you think is happening to Mrs Brown?
Q2. What action do you need to take?

Hyperglycaemia (Hyper = high, glyce = glucose and emia = blood) occurs when there is not enough insulin and the blood glucose level remains high. If there is no insulin produced, glucose is unable to enter the cells. Signs that may be observed in patients are thirst and hunger. As the blood glucose continues to be elevated, excess glucose is excreted in urine; however, as the level of glucose increases, the kidneys are unable to reabsorb the water and large amounts of urine are excreted and this condition is known as *polyuria* (Watkins et al., 2003). The patient may feel thirsty and possibly hungry, which may lead to dehydration and a fall in blood pressure (Fig. 11.2).

There are complications that may affect patients who are diagnosed as diabetics. Long-term diabetes is a chronic condition and poor control of blood glucose may affect other parts of the body – for example, the brain, heart, kidneys, peripheral extremities and eyes. Microvascular (thickening of the membrane in blood vessels) and macrovascular diseases may result in complications for a patient with diabetes. The organs in the body affected by microvascular disease are the eyes (retinopathy), the kidneys (nephropathy) and the peripheral nerves (neuropathy) and also the arteries of the cardiovascular system (heart). Patients who are

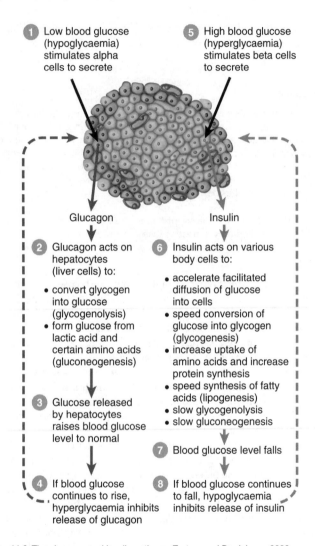

1 Low blood glucose (hypoglycaemia) stimulates alpha cells to secrete

5 High blood glucose (hyperglycaemia) stimulates beta cells to secrete

Glucagon

Insulin

2 Glucagon acts on hepatocytes (liver cells) to:

- convert glycogen into glucose (glycogenolysis)
- form glucose from lactic acid and certain amino acids (gluconeogenesis)

3 Glucose released by hepatocytes raises blood glucose level to normal

4 If blood glucose continues to rise, hyperglycaemia inhibits release of glucagon

6 Insulin acts on various body cells to:

- accelerate facilitated diffusion of glucose into cells
- speed conversion of glucose into glycogen (glycogenesis)
- increase uptake of amino acids and increase protein synthesis
- speed synthesis of fatty acids (lipogenesis)
- slow glycogenolysis
- slow gluconeogenesis

7 Blood glucose level falls

8 If blood glucose continues to fall, hypoglycaemia inhibits release of insulin

Fig. 11.2 The glucagon and insulin pathway. Tortora and Derrickson, 2009; reprinted with permission from John Wiley and Sons Inc.

diabetics may be at a greater risk of potentially developing all of the above complications (Marieb, 2009).

Type 1 and type 2 diabetic patients may be at risk of retinopathy as often they have had diabetes for several years before they are diagnosed. Blood vessels in the retina of the eye can become blocked, leaky or grow haphazardly. This damage prevents light from passing through to the retina and, if left untreated, can damage vision. Retinopathy affects the blood vessels supplying the retina – the 'seeing' part of the eye (Dunning, 2003). Keeping blood glucose, blood pressure and blood fat levels under control will help reduce the risk of the patient developing retinopathy; all diabetic patients are advised to have regular eye checks. The Diabetes National Service Framework (NSF) reiterates that everyone with diabetes must be offered screening for diabetic retinopathy (DH, 2003).

Patients who are diabetics may also develop nephropathy (kidney problems) because the kidneys are the organs that filter and clean the blood and get rid of any waste products (ketones) by producing urine. The kidneys regulate the amount of fluid including various salts in the body that help control our blood pressure. The kidneys start to fail because of damage to the small blood vessels; the vessels become leaky or, in some cases, stop working, making the kidneys work less efficiently. It is recommended that keeping blood glucose levels as near normal as possible and maintaining a blood pressure of 130/80 mmHg may help reduce the risk of developing kidney disease. One of the most important tests that can be performed is to test the patient's urine for protein (microalbuminuria), as the presence of albumin in the urine may indicate the first stage of kidney disease. If diabetic patients do not manage to control their diabetes, it is possible that they may be more susceptible to developing a urinary tract infection, as glucose in the urine provides the opportunity for bacteria to grow (Dunning, 2003).

Nerve damage (neuropathy) can also affect the nerves and flow of blood to the foot; therefore, the patients may not feel any pain or pressure on their feet. Because the patients may not feel pain, it is important that they are referred to a podiatrist who specialises in diabetes. While assisting patients with their hygiene needs, it provides an opportunity for observation of their skin for any signs of pressure points or cuts.

Areas such as an accident and emergency department or a coronary care unit may have patients who have been admitted and diagnosed as having an acute myocardial infarction (MI). Diabetes is known to impact on cardiovascular disease; as hormones are released and the blood sugar levels rise (Watkins et al., 2003). According to research by Malmberg (1997), patients with diabetes mellitus are more at risk after an acute MI and have a higher risk of mortality. Cardiac disease is a complication of diabetes and if the patients blood glucose levels are ≥11 mmol, they may be commenced on the Diabetes Mellitus Insulin Glucose Infusion in Acute Myocardial Infarction (DIGAMI) protocol. Patients commence on an intravenous insulin–glucose infusion for 24 hours. It is possible that the trust has adopted the DIGAMI protocol or has developed a trust protocol for patients who are diabetic and are admitted following an MI.

BLOOD SAMPLING

Taking a blood glucose sample will provide valuable information on a patient who is acutely unwell or on a patient with diabetes. Monitoring a patient's blood sugar provides an indication of how the body is controlling glucose metabolism. There are two ways of obtaining a blood sample; the first method is to take a sample of blood from the vein, which is then sent to the laboratory to be tested; or a simpler and quicker method is a capillary sample. A capillary sample of blood is obtained from the tiny blood vessels called *capillaries* that are near the surface of the skin on the finger.

How to obtain a blood sample

It is important that prior to the procedure the patient gives consent and that it is ensured that equipment is collected and available before taking the blood sample. In many healthcare settings, there is a blood glucose monitoring box that contains a disposable lancet, test strips, glucose monitoring device, gauze and a sharps disposal box. It is important to ensure before starting the procedure check that the glucose monitoring device has been calibrated within the last 24 hours and the same documented in the medical devices records (Fig. 11.3a and b). A high and low internal control test is completed and the expiry date on the test strips is also checked

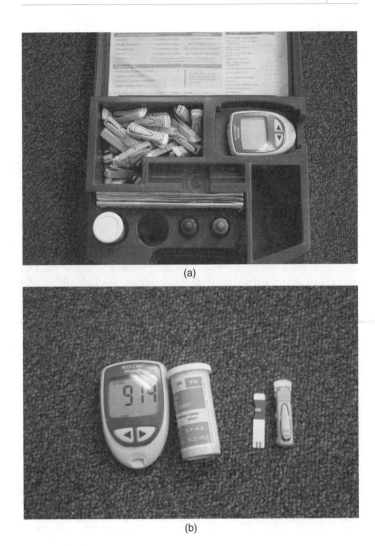

Fig. 11.3 (a) Glucose monitoring box and equipment and (b) glucose calibration kit (photographs).

prior to taking the blood sample and documented in the log book provided.

The next step is preparing the patients and making sure they are in a comfortable position. Wash your hands, put on a pair of gloves and a disposable apron. Please ask the patients to wash their hands prior to taking a sample of blood to ensure that their hands are as clean as possible, as any sugar on their fingers will result in a high reading (Higgins, 2008). Load the lancet as required and take a blood sample from the side of the patient's finger; remember to rotate the fingers and try not to use the index finger or thumb. If the blood sample is taken from the side of the finger, it is less painful for the patient (Dougherty and Lister, 2008). Ensure that the droplet of blood is sufficient to cover the test strip to ensure a correct reading; if not, the machine will not register the glucose level and the reading will be incorrect. Place the test strip into the blood glucose monitor and dispose of the lancet in the sharps box once the sample has been obtained. Apply gauze to the site and check that the puncture site has stopped bleeding; also make sure that the patient is comfortable. It is very important that the results are documented and if the blood glucose level is outside the normal range, discussion of the results must take place with a senior member of the healthcare team.

Cleaning and storage of glucose monitor

Once the blood sample has been taken, it is necessary to clean and store the glucose monitor in line with manufacturer recommendations, infection prevention procedures and clinical guidelines.

Practice point 11.2 Self-directed reflective study

Q1. Read through your policy or guidelines for glucose monitoring and reflect on your current practice.

Q2. How often do you check that your equipment is in line with your policy or guidelines and the manufacturer's recommendations?

It is also important when caring for patients who are critically ill, severely stressed or diagnosed with type 1 or type 2 diabetes to support assessment using the look, listen and feel approach.

Look at the patient and observe whether their respiratory rate is fast, slow, regular or irregular. Are they using their accessory muscle? Is their chest rising and falling equally? Are they pale and sweating or are they agitated, confused and restless? Check the vital signs chart and record what their blood pressure is. Is it high or low? Remember to record the blood glucose on the blood sugar chart if this is separate from the vital signs documentation.

Listen to what they are telling you as it may be important. Do they appear confused? Is their speech slurred and are they complaining of a headache? They may actually say they are not feeling well. They may tell you that they have not eaten their meal or that they are hungry. The patient may tell you that they have had an upset stomach or diarrhoea that has caused them to become unwell. While you are listening to them, you may be able to detect a pear drop or acetone smell from their breath.

Feel the patient's skin – is it dry, cold and clammy or is the patient flushed and sweating?

Applying a systematic approach to look, listen and feel, and monitoring the patient's blood glucose levels will provide important information. An altered blood glucose level may affect the patient's emotional and psychological perspective; therefore, reassurance and education form an important part of care delivery.

THE DIABETES NATIONAL SERVICE FRAMEWORK

The education of diabetic patients plays a vital role in self-care management programmes. In 2003, the Department of Health introduced 12 standards in the NSF. The aim is to improve the care and management of patients who have diabetes ensuring quality care throughout the United Kingdom (DH, 2003). In 1999, an expert Task Force was set up by the government to bring together the valuable work of patients and clinical organisations to develop self-management initiatives. The expertise of patients was recognised as an untapped resource in the effective management of chronic disease and it was recommended that 'Expert Patients' must become an integral part of the design and functioning of all local NHS services (DH, 2001). The Diabetes National Service Framework and National Institute for Health and Clinical Excellence (NICE) recommend education and self-management as an important factor in helping newly diagnosed patients to understand and manage their diabetes (DH, 2003; NICE, 2008). Lifelong intervention programmes such as Diabetes Education and Self-Management for Ongoing and Newly Diagnosed (DESMOND) diabetics are advocated by the Department of Health and NICE as being made available within the primary care setting or the acute trusts. All adults with diabetes are to receive high-quality care throughout their lifetime, including support to optimise the control of their blood glucose, blood pressure and other risk factors for developing the complications of diabetes.

The Department of Health has worked in collaboration with Diabetes UK to develop guidelines that will help improve patient's access to insulin pumps. Although not suitable for everybody, continuous subcutaneous insulin infusion or insulin pump therapy is a therapy for people with type 1 diabetes that is recommended by NICE as a treatment option (DH, 2007; NICE, 2008). The World Health Organisation (2005) states that diabetes is a chronic condition that ultimately places further demands on healthcare staff who need a core set of competencies for the 21st century to manage patients with chronic conditions.

CONCLUSION

Within this chapter, we have briefly discussed the anatomy and physiology of the pancreas and the production of insulin. Type 1 and type 2 diabetes have been discussed; however, in acute illness, monitoring and managing an abnormal glucose reading may be part of the current disease process. The metabolic process is affected by the blood glucose levels. The measurement and documentation of blood glucose is an essential part of monitoring a patient's vital signs. Abnormalities or any deviations in normal blood glucose levels may indicate signs that the patient is becoming acutely unwell. Any stressor on the body can result in an alteration in the body's metabolic response and therefore alter the patient's blood glucose level. Equally, patient's lifestyle factors such as rising obesity continue to have a detrimental effect on the rising number of young people diagnosed with diabetes (DH, 2003).

REFERENCES

Braun CA and Anderson CM (2007). *Pathophysiology: Functional Alterations in Human Health*. Baltimore, Lippincott Williams & Wilkins.

British Medical Association (2007). *Childhood Obesity*. London, BMA. www.bma.org.uk/ap.nsf/Content/ChildObesity.

Cowan T (1997). Blood glucose monitoring devices. *Clinical Nursing Practices*. Jamieson EM, McCall JM and Whyte LA (2002) 4th edn. London, Churchill Livingstone.

Department of Health (2001). *The Expert Patient: A New Approach to Chronic Disease Management for the 21st Century*. London, DH.

Department of Health (2003). *National Service Framework for Diabetes*. London, The Stationery Office.

Department of Health (2007). *Insulin Pump Services*: *Report of the Insulin Pumps Working Group*. www.dh.gov.uk/en/Publicationsandstatistics/ Publications/PublicationsPolicyAndGuidance/DH_072777.

Department of Health (2008). *Five Years On*: *Delivering the Diabetes National Service Framework*. London, DH. www.dh.gov.uk [Accessed 14th June 2009].

Dougherty L and Lister S (2008). *The Royal Marsden Hospital Manual of Clinical Nursing Procedures*. 7th edn. Oxford, Wiley-Blackwell.

Dunning T (2003). *Care of People with Diabetes. A Manual of Nursing Practice*. 2nd edn. Oxford, Blackwell Publishing Ltd.

Ferguson A (2005). Blood glucose monitoring. *Nursing Times* **101**(38), 28–29.

Higgins D (2008). Patient assessment Part 4 – blood glucose testing. *Nursing Times*. **104**(10), 24–25.

Malmberg K (1997). Prospective randomised study of intensive insulin treatment on long term survival after acute myocardial infarction in patients with diabetes mellitus. *British Medical Journal* **314**, 1512–1515. London, BMJ.

Marieb EN (2009). *Essentials of Human Anatomy and Physiology*. 9th edn. San Francisco, Pearson Benjamin Cummings.

McLeod A (2006). Intra- and extracranial causes of alteration in level of consciousness. In: *Neuroscience Nursing Assessment and Patient Management*, Woodward S (eds). London, Quay Books.

National Institute for Health and Clinical Excellence (2004a). *Type 1 Diabetes* www.nice.org.uk/CG015 [Accessed 4th March 2008].

National Institute for Health and Clinical Excellence (2004b). *Type 2 Diabetes*: *Prevention and Management of Foot Problems (CG10)*. www.nice.org.uk/nicemedia/pdf/CG010NICEguideline.pdf [Accessed 12th June 2008].

National Institute for Health and Clinical Excellence (2008). *Continuous Subcutaneous Insulin Infusion for the Treatment of Diabetes Mellitus*. www.nice.org.uk/nicemedia/pdf/TA151Guidance.pdf. [Accessed 12th June 2008].

Resuscitation Council UK (2006). *Advanced Life Support*. 5th edn. London, Resuscitation Council UK.

Seyle H (1956). *The Stress of Life*. 2nd edn. New York, Mcgraw–Hill.

Tortora GJ and Derrickson BH (2009). *Principles of Anatomy and Physiology*. 12th edn. Oxford, John Wiley and Sons Inc.

Tortora GJ and Nielsen MT (2009). *Principles of Human Anatomy*. 11th edn. Oxford, John Wiley and Sons Inc.

Watkins PJ, Amiel SA, Howell SL, and Turner E (2003). *Diabetes and its Management*. 6th edn. Oxford, Blackwell Publishing Ltd.

Waugh A and Grant A (2006). *Ross and Wilson Anatomy and Physiology in Health and Illness*. 10th edn. London, Churchill Livingstone.

Williams G and Pickup JC (2004). *Handbook of Diabetes*. 3rd edn. Oxford, Blackwell Publishing Ltd.

World Health Organisation (2005). *Preparing a Health Care Workforce for the 21st Century: The Challenge of Chronic Conditions*. World Health Organisation.

Record Keeping

INTRODUCTION

The Nursing and Midwifery 'Code' states that 'you must ensure that the healthcare record for the patient or client is an accurate account of treatment, care planning and delivery' (Nursing and Midwifery Council (NMC), 2008). A Health Record is defined in section 68 (2) Data Protection Act 1998 as *(a) 'consisting of any information relating to the physical or mental health or condition of an individual and (b) has been made by or on behalf of a health professional in connection with the care of that individual'*. Record keeping is a legal and professional requirement within healthcare practice and an integral part of monitoring the quality of patient care (Royal College of Nursing (RCN), 2008; NMC, 2009).

LEARNING OUTCOMES

By the end of this chapter, you will to be able to discuss the following:

❑ Government initiatives
❑ Nursing and Midwifery Council guidelines
❑ Legal and professional accountability
❑ The importance of recording vital signs

GOVERNMENT INITIATIVES

The Government has reinforced the importance of record keeping as a key element in providing quality service within the

Vital Signs for Nurses: An Introduction to Clinical Observations, First Edition.
Joyce Smith and Rachel Roberts.
© 2011 Joyce Smith and Rachel Roberts. Published 2011 by Blackwell Publishing Ltd.

National Health Service (NHS) and an essential component of risk management (DH, 1997; DH, 1998). In 2010, the Department of Health introduced 'Essence of Care Benchmarks', a nationally developed self-assessment benchmarking and audit tool that supersedes the previous 2001 benchmarks. There are twelve specific benchmarks that are patient focused and link to clinical governance. All twelve benchmarks are applicable in any health care setting, and record keeping is included as one of the benchmarks. The *Records Management: NHS Code of Practice* (DH, 2006) outlined a guide to the standards of practice required in the management of all NHS records. A collaborative approach to devise the guidance included representatives from the Department of Health, NHS Connecting for Health, GP practices, the NHS organisation and professional bodies. The guidance applies to all records including electronic or paper-based patient records. The important aspect identified within the standards is that information may be needed to support continuity of care and also to support evidence-based clinical practice.

To achieve its modernisation programme for healthcare systems including the National Health Service, all four countries within the United Kingdom have national programmes for introducing information and communications technology (ICT) (RCN, 2006). In England, 'NHS Connecting for Health' is responsible for delivering the information technology programme. Similar programmes are being introduced, for example, in Scotland – the *e-Health programme*; in Wales – *Informing health care* and in Northern Ireland – the *Health and Personal Social Services (HPSS) ICT programme* (Hutchinson and Sharples, 2006; RCN, 2006). The e-Health system refers to the range of information technology in healthcare and includes implementing an electronic patient record replacing traditional paper-based 'patients notes'. The plan is that every patient will have a single integrated electronic health record. The record will only be available via a secure network that only authorised users will be able to access; this will ensure that the patient record is accessible wherever a patient requires treatment or care.

The NHS Connecting for Health (2005) document *Information Governance* provides a framework for best practice that applies to the handling of patient information including standards to ensure that information is

- held securely and confidentially;
- obtained fairly and efficiently;
- recorded accurately and reliably;
- used effectively and ethically;
- shared appropriately and lawfully.

Hutchinson and Sharples (2006, p. 61) advocate the 'mnemonic' HORUS, which provides an appropriate reference point for nursing staff. A key message within *Information Governance* is to ensure the information recorded is accurate, legible and complies with the law. It is also a prerequisite that consent is obtained before sharing personal information. The recommendations and guidance in key government documents regarding record keeping are inline with the principles outlined by the NMC.

In 2009, the NMC updated the guidelines for record keeping, reiterating that the purpose of maintaining accurate records is to ensure that the patient receives seamless continuity of care between healthcare professionals. The guidelines apply equally to written records and computer-held records (NMC, 2009). The guidelines clearly state that records are factual, written as soon as possible after the event and any alterations or additions are dated and timed and include a signature. A healthcare professional records information on all aspects of care delivery; this involves numerous methods of recording including paper-based records, risks assessments, referrals, emails and electronic records. Best practice is advocated inline with NMC guidance that all records must be legible, accurate, signed with the practitioners designation, include the date, time and provide a chronological series of events using only agreed abbreviations (DH, 2010a). Bird and Robertson (RCN, 2010) state records should be written in black ink that is readable if photocopied and also be written in language that patients understand. If appropriate, the record may also be completed in collaboration with the patient. High-quality record keeping demonstrates that you have provided skilled safe care, and should not be viewed as optional but an integral part of care delivery.

The NMC also emphasises that documentation related to patient care must not include subjective statements, jargon or abbreviations (NMC, 2009). Dimond (2008) cautions against using abbreviations, but acknowledges that it is not always realistic in practice. Therefore, the recommendations are to only use the abbreviations that have been agreed by the trust or your employer. The original documentation in a patient's health record must not be altered or deleted with correction fluid. A straight line should be drawn through the incorrect record including the date, time and signature of the person making the alteration (NMC, 2009). This premise is reinforced by the Department of Health that any judgements or opinions recorded by a health professional, whether accurate or not, should not be deleted (DH, 2010b). Despite professional and government guidelines on the importance of record keeping, it appears that the consequences of poor record keeping are still evident.

Practice point 12.1

Review the following documentation and identify any abbreviations or potential inaccuracies within the care plan evaluation.

Mrs Cameron was SOB this am and mobilised UTT between two nurses. ~~On returning to bed, pt~~ took H_2O and diet orally. Vital signs are satisfactory. All cares given.

SN ERB

LEGAL AND PROFESSIONAL ACCOUNTABILITY

Record keeping should provide objective, accurate, current, comprehensive and relevant information concerning the assessment and care provided by healthcare professionals. Any aspects of the patient's records can be required as evidence before a coroner's court, a court of law or before the professional conduct committee of the NMC (NMC, 2009; Dimond, 2008). In order to clarify what is considered a legal document, Dimond (2008) reiterates that 'any documents requested by the court becomes a legal document'; for example, the patient's physiological observation chart and fluid balance chart may be requested as evidence by the courts.

Therefore, poor record keeping may impact on the validity of the healthcare professionals' records when they are required to give evidence. Equally, registered nurses are held accountable for their record keeping by the NMC. The NMC is the regulator of nurses and midwives, and in their 'Fitness to Practice' annual report 2008/2009 poor record keeping is one of the top three reasons that practitioners appear before the fitness to practice panel.

It is not only healthcare professionals who must demonstrate accurate records as part of their professional regulatory body but also the healthcare organisation that must have systems in place to ensure high-quality standards of record keeping. The National Health Service Litigation Authority (NHSLA) is a special health authority that administers the Clinical Negligence Scheme for Trusts (CNST). The scheme is voluntary; however, all the NHS trusts, foundation trusts and primary care trusts in England have joined the scheme. The CNST deals with all clinical negligence claims against the NHS trusts that have joined the scheme after 1995. There are seven core standards relating to clinical risk management. All trusts who join the scheme are assessed against the seven core standards.

If a claim is made against the NHS trust, they are the legal defendant but the NHLSA is responsible for meeting the costs of any claim. Standard four of the core standards relates to health records keeping and within the standard are three levels that trusts need to achieve. All trusts within the scheme must ensure that there is a risk management process in place to maintain the standards and quality of their paper and electronic health records (NHLSA, 2010). Recent initiatives by the Department of Health (2009a), National Institute for Health and Clinical Excellence (NICE, 2007) and the National Patient Safety Agency (NPSA, 2007) all advocate the importance of recognising and responding to the patients' vital signs, including the significance of accurate record keeping. The Audit Commission (1999), following a review of health records, advocated that record keeping forms part of an organisation's audit system. Clinical Governance was introduced in 1999 with the aim of reducing risk and ensuring a quality service for patients, and it holds organisations accountable for the quality of their services. Clinical Governance is now an integral part of risk management and audit is a key component. The National Institute for Health and Clinical Excellence describes audit as a process for quality improvement for patient care and outcomes through a systematic review of the care against explicit criteria and the implementation of change therefore as a cyclic process (NICE, 2007). Several NHS trusts have now included vital signs observation charts as part of the ward audit calendar.

RECORDING VITAL SIGNS

On admission to any healthcare environment, it is usually routine practice for patients to have their vital signs taken and recorded in either the case notes or on a physiological observation chart. NICE (2007) recommend that every patient admitted to an acute hospital must have the vital signs recorded, and although the guidelines are aimed at an acute setting the guidelines are relevant to all healthcare settings. The patients' vital signs must be recorded accurately on the observation chart and documented in the patients' notes or Kardex. The date, time and designation of the person taking and recording vital signs also need to be included. Documenting the patient's vital signs provides not only a base line of parameters but also a visual graph that displays the trends of each parameter. The patient's observation chart provides documentary evidence of the assessment, and therefore needs to be complete, accurate and legible. However, concerns have been raised that often vital signs are not recorded accurately. The National Patient Safety Agency (NPSA) over a one-year period in 2005 analysed 576 deaths and found that often there was incomplete and inadequate documentation that was illegible or unclear. The key themes that emerged included incomplete recording of the patient's vital signs and fluid balance charts. Early warning scores were not fully completed or calculated incorrectly and staff failed to record baseline observations or subsequent scores (NPSA, 2007). Beaumont et al. (2008) searched the National Reporting and Learning System (NRLS) that records patient safety incidents in England and Wales. The review consisted of 58 incidents that had not resulted in the patient's death. In 26 of the 58 incidents, there was a failure to recognise the implications of deteriorating vital signs and in 24 incidents no observations were recorded.

It is therefore important when taking and recording vital signs that a systematic approach is applied to your record keeping. Decisions made by healthcare professionals on the frequency of recording the vital signs must be documented in the care plan to ensure continuity of care. Each physiological observation that has been requested following the initial assessment must be included on the relevant charts. Failing to include all the vital signs that have been requested will result in inaccurate charts that will have not only consequences for the patient but also professional and legal implications regarding the care delivered. It is unacceptable and poor practice to omit vital signs that have been requested or in the judgement of the healthcare professional advocated as essential. For example, if only the patient's temperature is recorded, the observation chart is not only incomplete, but more importantly, there is also the potential to miss signs of deterioration. If an early warning scoring (EWS) tool is in place, this must be completed and scores calculated for each vital sign.

In response to the National Institute for Clinical Excellence (NICE, 2007) clinical guideline 50, the Department of Health introduced a framework for healthcare staff competencies, *Competencies for Recognising and Responding to Acutely Ill patients in Hospital* (DH, 2009b). A clear recommendation within the framework is that organisations must ensure that healthcare staff have the competences to accurately record and document vital signs. There is an assumption within the framework that healthcare staff will apply and possess certain generic competences and one example is record keeping (DH, 2009b).

Communication is essential when there is concern that the patient's vital signs are outside of their normal parameters or triggering an early warning score. NICE (2007) and the NMC (2009) reinforce the importance of good communication between healthcare professionals supported by evidence-based written information. The factors that contributed to a failure to respond to signs of deterioration included a breakdown in written communication (NPSA, 2007). The reasons that healthcare professionals are implicated in legal and professional issues are often related to a failure to maintain accurate records of patient care (NMC, 2009; Griffith and Tengnah, 2010). There is often no record of the date or time that care was provided and no record of the actions that the healthcare professional has taken. Poor record keeping may indicate poor care delivery (McGeehan, 2007) and there is a belief within the legal system that if care is not documented it did not happen (Wood, 2002).

CONCLUSION

In this chapter, government initiatives and professional guidelines on record keeping are highlighted including the legal and professional accountability of healthcare professionals in maintaining accurate records. The importance of recording and documenting the patient's vital signs including any action taken has been highlighted as crucial in recognising and responding to early signs of deterioration (NICE, 2007; NPSA, 2007; DH, 2009b). Poor record keeping has consequences for effective communication and ultimately effective patient care. By maintaining contemporaneous records, healthcare professionals demonstrate accurate record keeping and continuity of patient care.

REFERENCES

Audit Commission (1999). *Setting the Record Straight: A Review of Progress in Health Records Services.* www.audit-commission.gov.uk [Accessed 16th February 2010].

Beaumont K, Luettel D, and Thompson R (2008). Deterioration in hospital patients: early signs and appropriate actions. *Nursing Standard* **23**(1), 43–48.

Bird A and Robertson G (2010). *Documentation and Record Keeping.* London, RCN. www.rcn.org. [Accessed 8th February 2010].

Department of Health (1997). *Caldicott Report.* London, DH.

Department of Health (1998). *Data Protection Act.* London, DH.

Department of Health (2006). *Records Management NHS Code of Practice. Part 1.* London, Department of Health. www.dh.gov.uk [Accessed 11th August 2009].

Department of Health (2009a). *Records Management NHS Code of Practice. Part 2.* 2nd edn. London, Department of Health. www.dh.gov.uk [Accessed 15th January 2010].

Department of Health (2009b). *Competencies for Recognising and Responding to Acutely Ill Patients in Hospital.* http://www.dh.gov.uk/publications [Accessed 12th March 2010].

Department of Health (2010a). *Essence of Care 2010.* London, DH, The Stationery Office.

Department of Health (2010b). *Guidance for Access to Health Records Requests.* www.dh.gov.uk [Accessed 18th April 2010].

Dimond B (2008). *Legal Aspects of Nursing*. 5th edn. Essex, Pearson Education Limited.

Griffith R and Tengnah C (2010). *Ethics Foundations in Nursing and Health Care*. 2nd edn. Cheltenham, Nelson Thornes.

Hutchinson C and Sharples C (2006). Information governance: practical implications for record-keeping. *Nursing Standard* **20**(36), 59–64.

McGeehan R (2007). Best practice in record-keeping. *Nursing Standard* **21**(17), 51–55.

National Institute for Health and Clinical Excellence (2007). *Acutely Ill Patients in Hospital: Recognition and Response to Acute Illness in Adults in Hospital*. Guideline 50. London, NICE.

National Patient Safety Agency (2007). *Recognising and Responding Appropriately to Early Signs of Deterioration in Hospitalised Patients*. London, NPSA. www.npsa.nhs.uk [Accessed 15th April 2010].

NHS Connecting for Health (2005) *Health and Social Care Staff Members: What You Should Know About Information Governance*. www.connectingforhealth.nhs.uk/.../infogov/.../infogovleaflet.pdf [Accessed 12 November 2010].

NHS Litigation Authority (2010). *NHSLA Risk Management Standards For Acute Trusts, Primary Care Trusts and Independent Sector Providers of NHS Care*. www.nhsla.com/NR036C.../201011AcuteISPCT StandardsFINAL [Accessed 20th March 2010].

Nursing and Midwifery Council (2008). *The Code Standards of Conduct, Performance and Ethics for Nurses and Midwives*, p6. London, NMC.

Nursing and Midwifery Council (2009). *Record Keeping: Guidance for Nurses and Midwives*. London, NMC. www.nmc.org.uk [Accessed 15th April 2010].

Royal College of Nursing (2006). *e-Health. Putting Information at the Heart of Nursing Care*. London, RCN. www.rcn.org.uk [Accessed 12th May 2010].

Royal College of Nursing (2008). *RCN e-Health Programme. Policy Briefing 09/2008. Consent to Access, Share, and Create e-Health Records*. London, RCN. www.rcn.org.uk [Accessed 15th May 2010].

Wood C (2002). The importance of good record-keeping for nurses. *Nursing Times* **99**(2), 26–27.

Continuing Professional Development

INTRODUCTION

Continuing Professional Development (CPD) is a framework for lifelong learning that is integral to the government's plans for quality in the National Health Service (NHS) and is closely linked to clinical governance. Lifelong learning is inextricably linked to the government's wider agenda for developing healthcare staff with the knowledge and skills required for the 21st century (Department of Health (DH), 1999, 2000, 2001, 2003). For registered nurses and midwives, it is also a professional and legal obligation to meet the Nursing and Midwifery Council (NMC, 2009) Post-Registration Education and Practice (PREP) requirement.

LEARNING OUTCOMES

By the end of this chapter, you will be able to discuss the following:

❑ Professional and Government regulations
❑ Personal development plan
❑ Personal development record/portfolio

The Department of Health (DH, 2004c) framework for lifelong learning emphasises the importance of lifelong learning for everyone working in the NHS and states that 'continuing to update and extend knowledge and skills is an essential feature of maintaining competent professional practice'. Agenda for Change (AfC), a pay system, involving all healthcare staff except doctors, dentists and

Vital Signs for Nurses: An Introduction to Clinical Observations, First Edition.
Joyce Smith and Rachel Roberts.
© 2011 Joyce Smith and Rachel Roberts. Published 2011 by Blackwell Publishing Ltd.

senior managers was implemented within the NHS (DH, 2004a). A key strand of AfC was the National Health Service Knowledge and Skills Framework (NHS KSF) that links pay and progression to performance (DH, 2004b). The framework outlines the knowledge and skills required for every member of the workforce to deliver quality care to patients. The purpose of the NHS KSF is to promote equality, value diversity and develop all members of staff to ultimately meet the needs of the public (DH, 2004). The KSF has 30 dimensions and 6 core dimensions that are relevant to every post within the NHS. The six core dimensions include communication, personal and people development, health safety and security, service improvement, quality and equality and diversity. The remaining 24 dimensions are specific and are grouped into themes that may not relate to every post. Each dimension has four levels including indicators that identify what knowledge and skills are applicable. For example, the post outline will include the level and indicators that determine what knowledge and skills are required for the post (DH, 2004b). The KSF is a framework for a development review process that links organisational goals with individual goals to develop the knowledge and skills required to provide quality care. Healthcare staff employed in an NHS trust will be familiar with the annual review and appraisal system. However, in the private health sector or independent sector, there may be a different process – for example, an appraisal system or an annual meeting arranged with the line manager. A key component of the KSF is a requirement for all healthcare staff to have a personal development plan (PDP) that is discussed during the annual review process or appraisal system. A PDP is advocated as identifying and addressing the learning needs of individual members of staff that link to core skills and organisational goals for lifelong learning (DH, 2001, 2004b, 2004c).

All healthcare settings should provide a PDP for healthcare staff as a PDP is advocated as a useful tool to identify personal and professional development needs (DH, 2004b, 2004c; The Quality Assurance Agency (QAA), 2009). To demonstrate lifelong learning, registered nurses and midwives are required to develop a personal profile and professional portfolio of evidence (NMC, 2008). A PDP is a cyclic process that involves self-assessment, planning, doing,

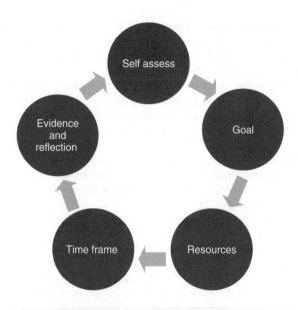

Fig. 13.1 Example of a cyclical personal development plan.

reviewing, evaluation and recording (Fig. 13.1) – for example, what do you need to know, are able to do, how will you develop the knowledge, skills and attitude that are required, what are the resources that are needed to achieve your goals and how will your achievement be demonstrated as evidence. Prior to developing a PDP, a self-assessment of the knowledge and skills you already possess against the knowledge and skills required to achieve your goal is needed. To complete a self-assessment, there are various helpful tools – for example, the Strengths, Weaknesses, Opportunities and Threats (SWOT) analysis tool (Table 13.1).

Once the self-assessment is completed, identify the short-term goals that will lead to developing long-term goals. Goals are expressed in terms that will enable you to determine whether they have been achieved; and therefore, goals must be specific, measurable, agreed and realistic including a timescale (SMART). Once your goals have been identified, the next step is to decide what action and resources will be required. Once you have fulfilled

Table 13.1 Example of a SWOT analysis related to recognising and caring for an acutely ill patient.

Strengths	Weaknesses
• Attended a Basic Life Support (BLS) course • Perform and record vital signs in daily practice • Knowledge of deviations of vital signs	• Limited experience in the assessment of an acutely ill patient • An understanding of altered pathophysiology during clinical deterioration
Opportunities	**Threats**
• Part of the trust policy to undertake the ALERT or AIM course • Protected study time • Places available on a recognised course	• Time to undertake the study day due to staffing levels • Balancing family commitments • Availability of a place on the course • Funding • Not passing the course

your goal, evidence must be provided to demonstrate that the goal has been achieved. The PDP needs to be completed before the appraisal meeting with the line manager, as this will provide a structured framework to discuss ongoing continuing professional development. The PDP must be signed and agreed by both the employee and the employer and is usually reviewed annually.

EXAMPLE OF PDP PROCESS

The first stage is self-assessment by asking 'What skills and knowledge do I now possess?' and then to decide, 'What skills and knowledge do I need to assess an acutely ill patient?' From the self-assessment, identify your short- and long-term goals. For example, a goal may state 'to be competent in the knowledge and skills required for recognising and responding to acutely ill patients'. The next stage requires identification of the resources that are available to achieve the goal. This may include support from your line manager, finance department, education and training department and access to the availability of a relevant course. The Department of Health (2009) advocates a framework for competences and suggests several one-day courses; two examples are the Acute Life-Threatening Events Recognition and Treatment (ALERT) or the Acute Illness Management (AIM) course. Once the resources have been identified to achieve the goal, the next stage is to arrange a place on a relevant course and identify a time frame for completion. The last stage is to produce the evidence to demonstrate the acquisition of knowledge and skills. This may include a certificate from the course, but also importantly, reflection on what has been achieved or learnt in the application of the course in clinical practice. To provide evidence and demonstrate further development, a record needs to be stored in either the format of a portfolio or a personal record of achievement.

PORTFOLIO

The Nursing and Midwifery Council is the regulatory body for nurses and midwives and PREP requirements are a professional standard and a legal requirement for their registration to be renewed (NMC, 2009). There are two separate PREP standards that are required for registration – the Post-Registration Education and Practice, PREP (practice) standard and the PREP (continuing professional development). During the 3-year period prior to the renewal of their registration, all registered nurses and midwives are required to complete 35 hours of learning relevant to their area of practice. All learning activities must be documented in a personal professional profile. Although there is no formalised way to develop a profile, the NMC has devised a template within the PREP handbook.

A portfolio, also known as a personal development record, has been identified as an excellent method of providing evidence that demonstrates continuing professional development (NMC, 2009) and has been adopted by unqualified staff following the introduction of the Knowledge and Skills Framework. Several academic courses may also require students to develop a portfolio specific to the aim and objectives of the module they have chosen. It is also a university requirement to provide students with an opportunity for PDP during their academic programme of study (QAA, 2009).

There is no prescriptive framework for developing a portfolio, but the PREP handbook provides a template to record learning activity; however, a portfolio provides an opportunity to create an individualised personal record of continuing development. If the employer does not provide a portfolio, a simple lever arch file is sufficient. An alternative is an e-portfolio, but whichever method is chosen, a range of evidence must be provided. Simply including certificates from study days or mandatory training days does not demonstrate what knowledge and skills have been developed or applied to your practice. It is important to structure the file systematically including an index page, as this will allow you to cross reference your evidence and provide easy access when locating relevant information. Divide your file into sections to create a structured approach – for example, the core dimensions of the Knowledge and Skills Framework may be considered a relevant format. Ideas for collecting evidence may include testimonials, pictures, significant events, teaching packages and reflection. Continuing professional development was valued by nurses in a study by Gould et al. (2007), who viewed continuing professional development as an intrinsic part of nursing that links theory to practice. Continuing professional development is an essential component of care delivery; therefore, the skills of self-awareness and reflection are invaluable (Bethell and Shepherd, 2008). Reflection is an integral part of your continuing professional development that demonstrates your problem-solving approach and critical thinking skills.

The importance of continuing professional development and lifelong learning has been reinforced by the Department of Health (DH) in its 'Acutely Ill Competency Framework'. The framework clearly advocates that 'healthcare staff working in any acute setting must have the education and training in monitoring, measurement and interpretation of vital signs and be assessed as competent' (DH, 2009, p. 7). This premise is reinforced by the National Institute for Health and Clinical Excellence (2007) and National Patient Safety Agency (2007). Several trusts are now assessing the knowledge and skills of healthcare staff in recognising and responding to acutely ill patients. The underpinning concept of the knowledge and skills required is an understanding of the related physiology in recording vital signs. Equally, the NMC (2008) clearly outlines the responsibility of practitioners to deliver care based on best practice and updated knowledge and skill.

CONCLUSION
In this chapter, the importance of personal development planning and creating a record of evidence through a paper-based or e-portfolio are reinforced as tools to demonstrate your continuing

professional development. If you are employed in the NHS trust, community or private health sector, you have a professional, legal and ethical responsibility to develop and maintain your knowledge and skills to provide quality patient care (DH, 2004b; NMC, 2008). Continuing professional development is seen as a tool for maintaining safe clinical practice and maintaining professional standards (NMC, 2008, 2009; Savage, 2008). It is possible that the relevance of a personal development record and portfolio is questioned; however, these are considered retrospective, current and prospective evidence of your personal, educational and professional achievement, providing the foundation for lifelong learning (Nixon, 2008).

REFERENCES

Bethell C and Shepherd R (2008). Continuing professional development and lifelong learning. In: *Portfolios in the Nursing Profession: Use in Assessment and Professional Development*, Norman K (ed). London, Quay Books.

Department of Health (1999). *A First Class Service: Quality in the New NHS*. London, The Stationery Office.

Department of Health (2000). *A Health Service of All the Talents: Developing the NHS Workforce*. London, DH. www.dh.gov.uk [Accessed 16th February 2008].

Department of Health (2001). *Working Together, Learning Together. A Framework for Lifelong Learning in the NHS*. London, Stationery Office.

Department of Health (2003). *Essence of Care: Patient-Focused Benchmarks for Clinical Governance*. NHS Modernisation Agency. London, DH.

Department of Health (2004a). *Agenda for Change*. London, DH. www.dh.gov.uk [Accessed 17th February 2008].

Department of Health (2004b). *The NHS Knowledge and Skills Framework (NHS KSF) and the Development Review Process*. London, DH. www.dh.gov.uk [Accessed 17th February 2008].

Department of Health (2004c). *Learning for Delivery: Making Connections Between Post Qualification Learning/Continuing Professional Development and Service Planning*. London, DH. www.dh.gov.uk [Accessed 12th February 2008].

Department of Health (2009). *Competencies for Recognising and Responding to Acutely Ill Patients in Hospital*. London, DH. http://www.dh.gov.uk/publications [Accessed 15th March 2008].

Gould D, Drey N, and Berridge EJ (2007). Nurses' experiences of continuing professional development. *Nurse Education Today* **27**, 602–609.

National Institute for Health and Clinical Excellence (2007). *Acutely Ill Patients in Hospital: Recognition and Response to Acute Illness in Adults in Hospital*. Guideline 50. London, NICE.

National Patient Safety Agency (2007). *Recognising and Responding Appropriately to Early Signs of Deterioration in Hospitalised Patients*. www.nspa.nhs.uk [Accessed 18th March 2008].

Nixon V (2008). Assessment. In: *Portfolios in the Nursing Profession*, Norman K (ed). London, Quay Books.

Nursing and Midwifery Council (2008). *The Code'. Standards of Conduct, Performance and Ethics for Nurses and Midwives*. London, NMC. www.nmc.org.uk [Accessed 12th April 2009].

Nursing and Midwifery Council (2009). *The Prep Handbook*. London, NMC. www.nmc.org.uk [Accessed 16th April 2009].

The Quality Assurance Agency for Higher Education (2009). *Personal Development Planning: Guidance for Institutional Policy and Practice in Higher Education*. Gloucester, QAA. www.qaa.ac.uk [Accessed 16th April 2009].

Savage S (2008). Maintaining professional standards. In: *Nursing Practice and Health Care. A Foundation Text*, Hinchliff, S, Norman S, and Schober J (eds). 5th edn. London, Hodder Arnold.

Reflective Practice

14

INTRODUCTION

Reflective practice is thought to be an important professional pastime for nurses. All nurses are encouraged to reflect upon their day-to-day activities within the workplace and their impact on patient care. It is mandatory for many nurses to maintain a portfolio of evidence that supports their post outline within the Agenda for Change (AfC) framework. It is especially important for registered nurses because of their professional body, the Nursing and Midwifery Council (NMC) and *The Code* NMC (2008).

In order to maintain up to date skills and knowledge, *The Code* NMC (2008, p. 4) states the following:

- You must have the knowledge and skills for safe and effective practice when working without direct supervision.
- You must recognise and work within the limits of your competence.
- You must keep your knowledge and skills up to date throughout your working life.
- You must take part in appropriate learning and practice activities, which maintain and develop your competence and performance.

According to the Royal College of Nursing (RCN, 2010), reflection is a key approach for nurses adopting the concept of lifelong learning. Undertaking reflective practice is one way of learning and

Vital Signs for Nurses: An Introduction to Clinical Observations, First Edition.
Joyce Smith and Rachel Roberts.
© 2011 Joyce Smith and Rachel Roberts. Published 2011 by Blackwell Publishing Ltd.

improving your clinical performance when undertaking clinical observations. Practising reflection is also a method in which nurses can become more self-aware about their role within the workplace and how their behaviour, interactions and communication with patients and colleagues can impact on providing high standards of care (Somerville and Keeling, 2004).

LEARNING OUTCOMES

By the end of this chapter, you will be able to discuss the following:

❑ What reflection is
❑ Different models of reflection
❑ A reflective case study using a model of reflection

WHAT IS REFLECTION?

Reflection is the 'act of contemplating prospective or retrospective events' (Kenny, 2003, p. 105). It is about how you examine your own behaviour or situation so that you can gain more insight and understanding about something. It is thought to be an active process that results in learning (Cooney, 1999). It has also been described as a 'problem solving' approach (Kenny, 2003, p. 105). Educationalists have developed many different models for reflection. Early published discussions around reflection identified two mechanisms of reflective practice; reflection in action and reflection on action (Schon, 1987). Reflection in action is often referred to as 'thinking on your feet' (Cooney, 1999), while reflection on action involves looking back on an experience and re-examining the situation. According to Cooney (1999, p. 1530), reflection 'enables nurses to examine their practice, before, during or after providing patient care'.

DIFFERENT MODELS FOR REFLECTION

There are several popular models of reflection described in literature such as Johns model (2000). From the author's experience, the two most popular models used for reflection are Gibbs cycle of reflection (Gibbs, 1988) and the Six Thinking Hats (DeBono, 2000). Let us have a look at these in more detail.

Johns model for structured reflection

This model can be used as a framework to reflect on a critical incident. By using a structured diary and a supervisor, the reflector can 'look into' the situation. When looking into the situation, think about your personal thoughts and feelings. Write these down in the diary. Then 'look out' of the situation by describing the circumstances of the situation and what you (and colleagues) were trying to achieve. Describe the reasons for responding the way you did and ask yourself if you responded in the best way and consider ethical issues. Reflect on internal factors such as stress of the situation; expectations and attitudes of others; time factors and whether or not it was a normal practice.

Gibbs reflective cycle

This model (Fig. 14.1) encourages you to describe the situation, analyse your feelings about the situation and then evaluate the

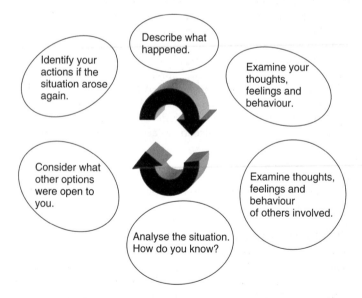

Fig. 14.1 Adapted Gibbs reflective cycle model.

situation, examining whether you would behave or act in the same way again, should the same situation were to arise again in the future.

Student nurses and health care assistants have demonstrated that reflection using Gibbs model has made a difference to them in practice through sharing their reflective experience in publications (Broderick, 2007; Wilding, 2008).

Practice point 14.1

Reflect on the following situation using Gibbs model.

Mrs Potterton is a 65-year-old woman who was admitted to a surgical ward with abdominal pain and constipation. Earlier this morning, Mrs Potterton went to theatre to have a growth removed from her bowel. Student nurse Hughes has been asked by SN Brook to perform her post-operative observations. Her previous BP recorded was 140/80 and pulse was 88 bpm. Student nurse Hughes goes to Mrs Potterton and informs her that she will be performing her clinical observations. She then proceeds to attach the Dinomap BP cuff to Mrs Potterton's left arm. She struggles to get the BP cuff around Mrs Potterton's arm. She decides to try and get the BP reading and presses the green button on the machine. The BP cuff inflates and then pops off Mrs Potterton's arm. Imagine you are student nurse Hughes, and reflect on this situation using Gibbs model of reflection and think about how you can learn from this situation.

Six Thinking Hats

Edward de Bono invented the Six Thinking Hats concept because he equates thinking and reflecting to 'putting our thinking caps on'. He calls thinking 'the ultimate human resource'. Traditionally, the person with the best argument wins it. But is winning the argument really useful for our personal and professional relationships? Issues with thinking relate to all the emotional feelings and the information and logic meshed within the situation. Within health care, there are often discussions that involve emotional feelings, diverse information and arguments about the best treatments for patients and staff. DeBono (2000) suggests that solutions or problems are more likely to happen when people discuss matters without their egos or emotions. It is not about winning an argument but about gaining balance and perspective about a situation. It is not about having the best personality or psychological makeup but about the focus on using appropriate behaviour. In his book, he tells the story of a man who painted one side of his car black and the other side of his car white. When asked why he painted the car this way he told his friends "Because it is such fun! I am amused after I have had an accident to hear the witnesses contradict themselves in court!" (DeBono, 2000, p. 2). As the saying goes, "There are two sides to every argument". DeBono encourages constructive thinking using his six thinking hats. Each hat is colour coded to represent a different way of thinking. If you look at the situation from the perspective of each coloured hat, then hopefully you will gain a more in-depth reflective perception of the situation. The six hats are coloured white, red, black, yellow, green and blue. Each

Table 14.1 Six Thinking Hats.

The white hat – provides information. Is neutral and objective	What information do you know? What information is missing? What questions should I ask? Whom should I ask? How can I get this information?
The red hat – provides feelings and emotions	How do I feel? How does the patient feel? What emotions do I feel? What emotions does the patient feel?
The black hat – provides caution and asks for care. Highlights weakness and risk	What judgement can be made in light of the facts? What policies and procedures are in place? Were these followed? What risks are there to the patient? What risks are there to me and my colleagues? What ethical considerations are there?
The yellow hat – provides optimism and positivity. Looks at the benefits	What is good about this situation? What are the benefits? What values are being expressed?
The green hat – provides creativity and new ideas, allows for growth and development	What ideas and solutions do we have? What alternative actions could we use?
The blue hat – provides control and organisation of thinking	What have we achieved so far? What have we reflected upon?

colour symbolises a thinking role. Let us look at these in more detail (see Table 14.1).

You can use the six thinking hats on your own or it can be used by a group of people during a meeting. There are some ground rules to using the technique. When using the thinking hats in a group meeting, only the chairperson can change the thinking hat. When using the hats, always start and finish with the blue hat. It will help outline the issues and also reflect on the solutions. Allow each member of the meeting to express their opinion through each hat but it is advised that each member be limited to a minute, before the chairperson moves the meeting forward. This will keep the meeting focused and reduce time wasting. It is important to remember that not all coloured hats are required when reflecting upon a situation. You can chose to use this model of reflection on your own or you can use it within your clinical team to gain different perspectives of the situation. It may be useful to have a facilitator to help keep the reflective debate constructive and professional and ensure that it takes place in a productive and respectful way.

Practice point 14.2

Mr Leonard is a 72-year-old man who has been undergoing a course of chemotherapy. It is dinner time and the staff on the ward start to distribute the meals and drinks. When you arrive at Mr Leonard's bed area, he takes a look at the meal and states that he does not feel like eating it and asks you to take it away. Using deBono's six thinking hats, consider the above situation and what you can do to get Mr Leonard to eat his meal.

The white hat – provides information. Is Neutral and objective	What information do you know? What information is missing? What questions should I ask? Whom should I ask? How can I get this information?
The red hat – provides feelings and emotions	How do I feel? How does the patient feel? What emotions do I feel? What emotions does the patient feel?

(continued)

Continued

The black hat – provides caution and asks for care. Highlights weakness and risk	What judgement can be made in light of the facts? What policies and procedures are in place? Were these followed? What risks are there to the patient? What risks are there to me and my colleagues? What ethical considerations are there?
The yellow hat – provides optimism and positivity. Looks at the benefits	What is good about this situation? What are the benefits? What values are being expressed?
The green hat – provides creativity and new ideas, allows for growth and development	What ideas and solutions do we have? What alternative actions could we use?
The blue hat – provides control and organisation of thinking	What have we achieved so far? What have we reflected upon?

You may find that you do not find any of the previous reflective models suited to your style of learning. You could always decide to develop your own like Peter Welsby, a charge nurse from Derbyshire. Peter Welsby (2007) developed his own model of reflection based on the REFLECT mnemonic that some nurses may prefer to use. REFLECT stands for

R = Research
E = Experience
F = Feelings
L = Learning
E = Evaluate
C = Continue
T = Teach

Research the situation or task. Know the rationale and reasoning for a task and how to perform it – for example, correctly performing clinical vital signs such as blood pressure, pulse, temperature and respiration rates. There is no point in performing clinical observations if you do not know the difference between normal and abnormal parameters or how to use the equipment correctly.

Experience at undertaking the task will help you achieve best practice and competence. Can you use the experience of others to assist your learning as well as improve your own skills – for example, practicing manual and electronic blood pressure under the supervision of more experienced staff.

Feelings about the situation. Do you feel uncomfortable, out of your depth, insecure or confident and competent? Why do you have these feelings and what action do you need to take? For example, a lot of nurses have lost the skill to use the manual sphygmomanometer and stethoscope and feel nervous about using it. The action required to overcome this fear is to acknowledge these feels and discuss with a senior member of staff to identify it as a area within your PDP.

Learning from the situation or task. What have you learnt and how do you feel? Can you perform this skill any better or differently? What have you learnt about yourself – for example, completing a literature search relating to manual blood pressures or reading the hospital guidelines on performing the procedure and then practicing the skill on colleagues and patients.

Evaluate research, experience, feelings and learning and decide whether you are confident as well as competent in the situation or task. Do you need to focus on one aspect of the RESPECT – for example, performing manual blood pressure and then discussing with a senior member of staff whether it was performed correctly and how to troubleshoot problems encountered during the task.

Continue to complete the task or deal with the situation without assistance. If you feel unsure, think about returning to R, E, F, L or E.

Teach the skill to someone else because you have researched, experienced and examined your feelings, learnt and evaluated your skills and are now are able to pass your knowledge and skills on to others.

CONCLUSION

According to Cowan (2003), using reflective practice is the precursor to change. Reflection should be embedded into your professional behaviour so that you can provide high-quality care to your patients. By reflecting on your current practice of performing clinical skills you will change. You will change because you will start to view the task or situation from different view points. Hopefully, you improve your clinical practice and therefore provide better quality of care to your patients.

REFERENCES

Broderick L (2007). A language barrier. *British Journal of Healthcare Assistants* **1**(7), 322.

Cooney A (1999). Reflection demystified: answering some common questions. *British Journal of Nursing* **8**(22), 1530–1534.

Cowan T (2003). Reflection is the precursor to change. *Journal of Wound Care.* **12**(1), 3.

DeBono E (2000). *Six Thinking Hats*. London, Penguin.

Gibbs G (1988). *Learning by Doing: A Guide to Teaching and Learning Methods*. Oxford, Oxford Further Education Unit, Oxford Polytechnic.

Johns C (2000). *Becoming a Reflective Practitioner: A Reflective and Holistic Approach to Clinical Nursing, Practice Development and Clinical Supervision*. Oxford, Blackwell Publishing Ltd.

Kenny L (2003). Using Edward deBono's six hats game to aid critical thinking and reflection in palliative care. *International Journal of Palliative Nursing* **9**(3), 105–112.

Nursing and Midwifery Council (NMC) (2008). *The Code*. www.nmc.org [Accessed March 2008].

Royal College of Nursing (RCN) 2010. *Principles for Inclusive Practice.* http://www.rcn.org.ok/development/practice/social_inclusion/principles [Accessed January 2010].

Schon DA (1987). *Educating the Reflective Practitioner*. London, Temple Smith.

Somerville D and Keeling J (2004). A practical approach to promote reflective practice within nursing. *Nursing Times* **100**(12), 42–45.

Welsby P (2007). Developing a clinical reflection model. *Nursing Times* 4th January 2007. http://www.nursingtimes.net.

Wilding PM (2008). Reflective practice: a learning tool for student nurses. *British Journal of Nursing* **17**(11), 720–724.

Conclusion and Multiple Choice Questions

15

As you have read each chapter in this book, the importance of infection prevention including legal and ethical principles has underpinned the knowledge and skills required by you to undertake and monitor a patient's vital signs. The importance of a systematic approach to the patient's assessment has been reiterated in each chapter including the importance of the look, listen and feel approach. Record keeping has emerged not only as a legal requirement but also as a key element in recognising, responding and communicating the patient's vital signs to members of the multidisciplinary team.

Government initiatives and guidelines have reinforced the need to ensure that every member of the healthcare team who performs and monitors vital signs is educated, trained and assessed as competent (NICE, 2007; NPSA, 2007; DH, 2009). The role of all healthcare staff is to maintain the patient's dignity and treat each patient with respect, irrespective of race, ethnicity, beliefs or age (NMC, 2009; Equality Act, 2010). The aim and theme throughout the book is to empower your knowledge in performing and recording a patient's vital signs. In addition, the early recognition and importance of responding in a timely manner to the early signs of a patient's deterioration are reiterated as integral in assessing an acutely ill patient. Continuing professional development is a prerequisite for providing evidence-based care and maintaining professional standards. To reinforce your knowledge, a set of multiple choice questions based on each chapter has been devised. The questions are related to all aspects of a patient's vital signs, and

Vital Signs for Nurses: An Introduction to Clinical Observations, First Edition.
Joyce Smith and Rachel Roberts.
© 2011 Joyce Smith and Rachel Roberts. Published 2011 by Blackwell Publishing Ltd.

it is hoped that you find this a fun way to check how you have developed and reinforced your knowledge.

MULTIPLE CHOICE QUESTIONS (MCQ)

Completion of the multiple choice questions will reinforce your knowledge from reading the chapters throughout the book.

Infection Control

What is the body's first line of defence?
(a) Cilia
(b) Skin
(c) Nose
(d) Eyes
(e) Respiratory tract

How are micro-organisms spread?
(a) Direct contact
(b) Airborne
(c) Bloodborne
(d) Indirect contact
(e) All of the above

How many levels are there in the chain of infection?
(a) 3
(b) 4
(c) 6
(d) 5

How many steps are there in the hand washing procedure?
(a) 5
(b) 4
(c) 3
(d) 7

Respiratory

The respiratory system consists of
(a) the lungs
(b) diaphragm
(c) trachea
(d) intercostals muscles
(e) all of the above

The normal respiratory rate is
(a) 6–10 bpm
(b) 12–20 bpm
(c) 20–24 bpm
(d) 18–24 bpm

When we breathe out it is called
(a) inhalation
(b) input
(c) expiration
(d) hyperventilation

The breathing patterns are
(a) tachypnoea
(b) dyspnoea
(c) Cheyne–Stoking
(d) all of the above

How long should it take to wash your hands?

(a) 10–15 minutes
(b) 8–12 seconds
(c) 15–30 seconds
(d) 20–35 seconds

The cardiovascular system
The blood leaves the heart at the
(a) left atrium
(b) left ventricle
(c) right ventricle
(d) right atrium
(e) all of the above

Name the three layers of the heart.
(a) Endocardium
(b) Pericardium
(c) Myocardium
(d) Epithelia

The blood pressure consists of

(a) the systolic
(b) the diastolic
(c) mean pressure
(d) all of the above

The normal pulse rate is

(a) 40–50 bpm
(b) 60–100 bpm
(c) 100–120 bpm
(d) 35–55 bpm

The most sensitive indicator that the patient is becoming unwell is
(a) the pulse
(b) the blood pressure
(c) the respirations
(d) the temperature

Early warning score
What score triggers a response?

(a) 2
(b) 4
(c) 3
(d) 5
(e) 1

What does AVPU mean?

(a) A diagnosis
(b) A test
(c) Conscious level
(d) Sleep patterns

The pulse above the systolic blood pressure is called
(a) peacock sign
(b) pigeon sign
(c) seagull sign
(d) magpie sign

What causes an inaccurate reading on a pulse oximeter?
(a) Nail varnish
(b) False nails
(c) Poor circulation
(d) Bright lights
(e) All of the above

Pain

The meninges are

(a) dura mater
(b) arachnoid
(c) pia mater
(d) all of the above

The body produces natural analgesics called
(a) endocrinology
(b) endorphins
(c) nociceptors
(d) encephalin

Record keeping

Written documentation should be recorded in
(a) blue
(b) green
(c) black
(d) red
(e) any colour

Documentation needs to be

(a) dated
(b) signed
(c) legible
(d) timed
(e) all of the above

Nutrition

Which tool assesses nutritional status?
(a) Risk assessment tool
(b) Waterlow tool

Communication

What are the barriers to communication?
(a) Anger
(b) Deafness
(c) Fear
(d) Anxiety
(e) All of the above

An acronym for communication is
(a) SOLER
(b) SBAR
(c) RBS
(d) HBOS

Diabetes

The normal level for blood sugar is
(a) 6–8 mmol
(b) 3–5 mmol
(c) 4–7 mmol
(d) 5–9 mmol

If the blood sugar is low the condition is called
(a) hyperglycaemia
(b) hypoglycaemia
(c) hypertension
(d) hypotension

Urine

The kidneys

(a) filter blood
(b) remove waste

(c) MUST tool
(d) Diet tool

How much water does the body need daily?
(a) 1–2 l
(b) 2–4 l
(c) 4–5 l
(d) 2–3 l

A normal BMI is

(a) <19
(b) >30
(c) 25–30
(d) 19–25

The best route for nutrition is

(a) enteral
(b) parenteral
(c) oral
(d) nasogastric

Legal and ethical
Unqualified healthcare staff are

(a) responsible
(b) accountable
(c) professionally accountable
(d) not accountable

(c) control fluid
(d) regulate electrolytes
(e) all of the above

How do we calculate urine output?
(a) Weigh the urine
(b) Patient's weight
(c) Fluid intake
(d) Urine output
(e) Fluid output

The hormones produced by the kidneys are
(a) renin
(b) vitamin D
(c) erythropoietin
(d) prostaglandins
(e) aldosterone

How much blood from the heart do the kidneys need to produce urine?
(a) 50%
(b) 40%
(c) 25%
(d) 20%

Temperature
Where do we measure the temperature?
(a) Mouth
(b) Ear
(c) Armpit
(d) Forehead
(e) All of the above

What are the ethical principles?

(a) Justice
(b) Beneficence
(c) Non-maleficence
(d) Autonomy
(e) All of the above

Valid consent is

(a) written
(b) verbal
(c) implied
(d) all of the above

Professional development

Developing your knowledge and skills is a key element in

(a) safe and effective care
(b) competence
(c) clinical governance
(d) personal development
(e) all of the above

A normal temperature is

(a) 36.8°C
(b) 39.0°C
(c) 38.5°C
(d) 37.0°C

The amount of insensible loss is

(a) 200 ml
(b) 100 ml
(c) 800 ml
(d) 500 ml
(e) 50 ml

Reflection

A model of reflection is

(a) Gibbs
(b) Johns
(c) Driscoll
(d) deBono
(e) All of the above

REFERENCES

Department of Health (2009). *Competencies for Recognising and Responding to Acutely Ill Patients in Hospital.* http://www.dh.gov.uk/publications.

Equality Act 2010. www.legislation.gov.uk/ukpga/2010/15/pdfs/ukpga_20100015_en.pdf.

National Institute for Health and Clinical Excellence (2007). *Acutely Ill Patients in Hospital: Recognition and Response to Acute Illness in Adults in Hospital.* Guideline 50. London, NICE.

National Patient Safety Agency (2007). *Recognising and Responding Appropriately to Early Signs of Deterioration in Hospitalised Patients.* www.nspa.nhs.uk [Accessed 18 th March 2008].

Nursing and Midwifery Council (2009). *Guidance for the Care of Older People.* London, NMC.

Glossary of Terms

Accessory muscles: Collective name for the muscles that support breathing

Acute pain management: The treatment of pain associated (linked to) with tissue damage

Agenda for Change: Introduced by the Government as a national pay system where all members of the healthcare team are banded

Alveoli: Air sac within the lung where gas exchange takes place

Anaerobic metabolism: The process of metabolism but without oxygen

Anaphylactic shock: An overwhelming severe reaction to something – for example, fish products or drugs. Causes the airways to swell, which affects breathing. Can be fatal if untreated

Aorta: The largest artery in the body that supplies oxygenated blood for circulation

Arachnoid: This is the middle layer of the meninges that protects the brain and spinal cord and is likened to look like a spider's web

Arterioles: The smallest sized arteries

Audible information: Data or information gathered through listening

AVPU: A quick assessment of the patient's conscious level – Alert, Voice, Pain, Unconscious

Axon: Neuron process that carries the impulses away from the nerve cell body

Bicuspid valve: Valve found inside the heart

Bile: Green fluid product that is produced by the liver to aid in the emulsification of fats

Vital Signs for Nurses: An Introduction to Clinical Observations, First Edition.
Joyce Smith and Rachel Roberts.
© 2011 Joyce Smith and Rachel Roberts. Published 2011 by Blackwell Publishing Ltd.

Blood pressure: Also known as BP. This is the amount of pressure exerted on the wall of the arteries by the amount of blood flowing through them. There are two components measured in BP. These are systolic and diastolic pressure.

Systolic is measured when the heart contracts and diastolic when the heart relaxes

Bronchi: These are the two main airway branches of the lungs. They are called the right and left bronchi

Bronchioles: The right and left bronchi subdivide into smaller airway branches called bronchioles

Capillaries: Tiny blood vessels

Capillary refill: Indicates how well the circulating blood volume is in our body

Cardiogenic shock: Cardiac-induced shock

Central nervous system (CNS): Consists of the brain and the spinal cord

Cerebrospinal fluid: Clear watery fluid that covers the brain and the spinal cord contained in the subarachnoid space

Cheyne–Stoke: Irregular breathing that is characterised by periods of apnoea

Cilia: Hair-like projections found in the respiratory airways

Commensal microbes: Microbes that live in specific parts of the body and do not cause harm to it – for example, bacteria in the bowel

Competent: Someone who has been assessed as skilled and knowledgeable in a task or skill and is deemed credible and accomplished within the specified clinical area by an assessor

Consciousness level: Level at which the brain is functioning. Best level is to be alert and orientated; worst level is to be unconscious

Cyanosis: Blue, dusky coloured skin that signifies depletion of oxygen

DH: Department of Health, which is the United Kingdom government department responsible for health regulations and policy

Diastolic: A component of the blood pressure. This is the phase where the heart's ventricles relax following contraction

Digestive enzymes: Proteins that will cause a catalytic reaction in digestion

DKA: Diabetic ketoacidosis where the blood glucose of the body is so high that it may become life threatening

Dura mater: Thickest and outermost of the three meninges surrounding the brain and the spinal cord

Dust: Dead skin and dirt that settle on surfaces and collect as dust

Duty of care: You must take reasonable care to avoid acts or omissions, which you can reasonably foresee would be likely to injure your patient

Dyspnoea: An increase in the respiratory rate that is greater than normal

Early Warning Score (EWS): A tool that calculates physiological scores and is an early predictor of physiological deterioration

Electrolytes: Sodium, potassium, magnesium and phosphate are some of the major substances, which when dissolved in the blood have an electrical charge

Epidural space: This space is outside the dura mater (the outer layer of the meninges) where anaesthetists will insert a catheter to provide pain relief

Expiration: The last part of the cycle of respiration. The breathing out phase

Extracellular: Extra means outside; therefore, outside the cellular space

Filtration: The removal of particles from the blood via a filter (semipermeable membrane)

General Medical Council (GMC): Governing body that regulates doctors

Glomerular filtration capsules: Found in the kidneys as part of the nephron

Glycogenesis: The process of food being broken down into sugars called glycogen

Glycogenolysis: The breakdown of glycogen (a form of sugar) which is used by the body to make energy

Gurgling: A sound made when there is fluid blocking the airways

Health care acquired infection (HCAI): Collective term for infections that have been caught through health care related contact

Homeostasis: The body in a stable state of equilibrium

Homoiothermic: Normal body temperature

Humidification: The use of heat and water to moisturise the airways and the lungs

Hypercarbia: High levels of carbon dioxide

Hyperglycaemia: High levels of glucose in the blood

Hypertension: High blood pressure that is not normal for the person's age and health

Hyperthermia: High body temperature

Hypervolaemia: High volumes of fluid in the body

Hypoglycaemia: Low levels of glucose in the blood

Hypotension: Low blood pressure that is not normal for the person's age and health

Hypothalamus: Found in the brain and controls the activities of the endocrine system and the levels of hormones

Hypothermia: Low body temperature

Hypovolaemia: Low volumes of fluid in the body

Hypovolaemic shock: Shock induced by lack of fluid

Hypoxia: Low levels of oxygen

Infection Prevention: Government-led strategy to reduce and prevent the spread of infection

Inferior vena cava: The lower part of the vena cava vein that carries deoxygenated blood

Inspiration: The active phase of breathing where the act of breathing in air causes the contraction of the intercostal muscles and diaphragm and expands the lungs

Interstitial: The space between the cells/tissues and the blood vessels

Intracellular: 'Intra' means within or inside; therefore, inside the cells

Liver: A large gland in the body that is responsible for many processes of metabolism. It controls glucose levels and production of hormones and vitamins

Mental Capacity Act: Act of Parliament to protect vulnerable adults who are unable to consent in the United Kingdom

Metabolic rate: The rate at which energy is released from the cells within the body

Metabolism: The total amount of chemical reactions that occur in the body to provide energy or to make substitute substances

Nephron: Part of the kidney that contains the glomerular capsule and collecting tubes

Nerve cell: One of the basic functional units of the nervous system

Nervous system: An extensive network of cells that are specialised in carrying information in the form of nerve impulses to and from all parts of our body

Neurogenic shock: Nervous system-stimulated shock

Neuropathy: The process where a nerve degenerates and impacts on nerve and body function – for example, diabetic neuropathy is associated with diabetes

Neurotransmitter: A chemical substance released from nerve endings to transmit impulses across synapse to other structures including nerves

NICE: National Institute for Health and Clinical Excellence. A United Kingdom Government-funded think tank that provides the best evidence for clinical practice via experts in their clinical fields

Nociception: The conduction of pain

Nociceptive fibres: Nerve fibres that are responsible for the transmission of pain

NPSA: National Patient Safety Agency – Government body that regulates health and safety within the NHS

Nursing and Midwifery Council (NMC): Governing body of nurses in the United Kingdom

Oxygen saturations: The amount of oxygen saturated within the blood and measured using pulse oximetry or taking a sample of blood

Pancreas: Large gland in the body that functions to control blood glucose by releasing insulin and aids in the digestion of food by the release of pancreatic enzymes

Pathogenic microbes: Microbes that live in the body but cause harm

Peak expiratory flow rate (PEFR): The maximum volume of one breath, often recorded from the best of three attempts

Pia mater: The inner layer of the meninges that covers the brain and the spinal cord

Pneumothorax: Air in the pleural cavity often referred to as a collapsed lung

Point of Care: The patient's immediate environment (zone) where contact or treatment is taking place

Poor perfusion: Reduced blood and oxygen supply to cell tissue within the body

Pulse: A palpable rhythmic beat in the arteries that can be felt using a finger. This rhythmic beat corresponds to the contraction of ventricles in the heart

Pyrexia: A temperature that is above 37.5°C

Reabsorption: Where substances are absorbed back into the body

Respiration rate: The rate at which a person breathes in and out. Respiration is made up of two phases: inspiration and expiration

Secretions: The release of fluid – for example, vomit and sputum

Sensory information: Information gathered and processed by the body using the senses (visual, touch, taste and smell)

Septic shock: Triggered by trauma or infection, this type of shock acts on systemic vascular resistance (SVR) of blood vessels, causing them to become more permeable and vasodilated. This allows fluid and volume to leak out into the interstitial space, which causes severe hypotension. This lack of BP then has an adverse effect on major organs

Spinal cord: Part of the central nervous system enclosed in the vertebral column comprising of nerve cells and bundles of nerves connecting all parts of the body with the brain

Statute: Statute Law and legislative act by the Government

Stridor: A harsh, shrill sound that is produced during respiration when there is an upper airway obstruction

Subarachnoid space: This is the space between the pia and arachnoid layers of the meninges. This contains cerebrospinal fluid. This is the fluid that is removed during the procedure of lumbar puncture

Subdural space: This is the space between the arachnoid and dura mater layers of the meninges

Superior vena cava: The upper part of the vena cava vein that carries deoxygenated blood

Systolic: Part of BP. The phase where the heart's ventricles contract to pump the blood out of the ventricles into the lungs and the rest of the body

Tachypnoea: Fast respiration rate that is abnormally high for a person

Temperature: Measures the amount of heat being produced by the body to maintain cell functions. How hot or cold a person is may indicate abnormal function or infection

Thalamus: Mass of grey matter in the diencephalon of the brain

The NHS KSF Framework: A framework of development and career progression for healthcare staff linked to PDPs

Thermometer: A tool used to measure the body temperature

Thorax: Another term for the chest. It is the hole within the chest that contains and protects a number of major organs that include the oesophagus, heart and lungs. The chest is held together by the diaphragm, sternum, ribs and thoracic spine

Tidal volume: The amount of air you breathe in and out of your lungs in one breath

Tricuspid valve: The valve that links the right atria of the heart to the right ventricle. 'Tri' means three. It opens to allow blood to drain into the ventricle and closes to prevent blood draining, but allows the right atrial chamber to start filling with blood again

Uraemia: High levels of urea and creatinine in the blood. Urea is the waste product of protein and normally is excreted by the body through the kidneys in the form of urine. However, if the body is unable to control the levels of urea and creatinine, then these toxic levels may cause nausea and vomiting. A person may complain of a headache and may even start to fit

Urethra: The channel leading from the bladder through which urine is expelled from the body. The length of the urethra varies in males (18 cm) and females (3.5 cm)

Urinate: The act of passing urine, commonly known as 'having a wee'. Also known as micturition

Urine output: The amount of urine measured. Ideally, 0.5 ml/kg to 1 ml/kg per person

UTI: Urinary tract infection

Vascular: Refers to a collection of blood vessels

Vasoconstriction: Where the diameter (lumen) of the muscle in the blood vessels shorten or shrink (constrict) to make the overall diameter of the blood vessel decrease

Vasodilatation: Where the diameter (lumen) of the muscle in the blood vessels stretch (dilate) to make the overall diameter of the blood vessel increase

Vasomotor: Vasomotor nerves control the changes in the size of the blood vessels. The vessels will either increase or decrease the size of the muscles within the blood vessel wall

Venules: The smallest of the veins which collect blood from the capillaries

Vicarious liability: A contract of employment; the employer accepts responsibility for the employee if they work within the policies and guidelines

Visual information: Information gathered and processed by the brain that has been obtained through sight and observation

Answers to Practice Points and Multiple Choice Questions

CHAPTER 1

Practice point 1.1

Q1. Although you have been on a venepuncture course within the trust or attended a course funded by your employer, you have not completed the supervised number required. Therefore, you should refuse to take the blood unsupervised. If you take the patient's blood, you are working outside of the guidelines identified by your employer and the course aims. If you cause any harm to the patient, they may bring a case of negligence against you and your employer.

Q2. Legally you are held responsible and accountable for your actions, if you work outside of your level of competence. Vicarious liability may also be called into question if you have failed to work within your employers' policy and guidelines.

Practice point 1.2

Take time out to consider how the patient gives consent to any intervention or procedure. Make notes in the box below.

Consent	Verbal	Implied	Written
Clinical observations	✓	✓	
Bed bath	✓	✓	
Venepuncture	✓	✓	
Medication	✓	✓	

(continued)

Vital Signs for Nurses: An Introduction to Clinical Observations, First Edition.
Joyce Smith and Rachel Roberts.
© 2011 Joyce Smith and Rachel Roberts. Published 2011 by Blackwell Publishing Ltd.

Continued

Urine sample	✓	✓	
Operation/procedure	✓		✓
Discuss treatment with a relative. You must have the patient's consent before disclosing any information	✓		✓
Discuss information over the telephone. You must have the patient's consent before disclosing any information	✓		✓

Practice point 1.3

Q1. John has told you in confidence; therefore, you must respect his wishes and maintain patient confidentiality.

Q2. What ethical issues do you think may emerge from this situation?

Points to consider: Conflict of interest. John is an adult; therefore, try to encourage John to talk to his parents. Offer support and advice on the services available.

CHAPTER 2

Practice point 2.1

1. Remove liquid gels from the environment.
2. Provide plenty of access to liquid soap, sinks and paper towels.
3. Encourage visitors to limit visits unless absolutely necessary to reduce exposure and risk of cross infection.
4. Verbally inform all staff, visitors and patients to wash hands using liquid soap and water.
5. Use signs to reinforce good hand hygiene.

6. Apply Aseptic Non Touch Technique (ANTT) principles in clinical areas.
7. Use gloves and aprons to protect clothing and cross infection if in direct patient contact.
8. Nurse patients with diarrhoea in a side room if possible and ensure that the door is closed at all times.
9. Liaise with the Infection Control team.

Practice point 2.2

Clinical activity	Sterile gloves	Non-sterile gloves	No gloves
Washing the patient's hands and face		✓	✓
Emptying the urinary catheter		✓	
Aspiration of PEG feeding line and changing feed	✓		
Changing a leg ulcer wound dressing	✓		
Cleaning and changing a stoma bag		✓	
Cleaning up vomit that has come in contact with the bed clothes		✓	
Emptying a urinal full of urine		✓	
Emptying a commode full of urine and faeces		✓	
Changing the dressing around a peripheral venflon site	✓		
Changing the dressing around a tracheostomy stoma site	✓		
Assisting the awake patient to brush their teeth		✓	✓
Providing eye care to the unconscious patient		✓	

Practice point 2.3

Clinical activity	No apron required	Sterile apron	Non-sterile apron
Bed bathing a patient			✓
Changing sheets on a bed			✓
Giving out meals			✓
Cleaning a bed area from a discharged patient			✓
Answering the telephone	✓		
Changing a stoma bag			✓
Recording physiological observations			✓
Cleaning a drip stand			✓

Practice point 2.4

1. First, make a visual risk assessment of the situation and ensure that the elderly gentleman is treated with dignity and respect, ensuring that he does not become further at risk of a slip, trip or fall. Take him to a private area to wash and change. He will be extremely embarrassed and will require understanding and support from the staff about the situation.
2. Make a visual risk assessment of the community clinic waiting room and remove other waiting patients away from the faecal matter to ensure that no one becomes at risk of a slip, trip or fall. If possible, use another room as a waiting area and podiatry. Once the area is isolated, staff can then gather cleaning materials to decontaminate the area.
3. Staff can refer to their local guidelines for following decontamination policy and ensure that they use PPE such as aprons, gloves and clinical waste disposal equipment.

CHAPTER 3

Practice point 3.1

Q1. The observations to be performed depend on what equipment you have available, but at a minimum, the respiratory rate, rhythm and depth need to be done. Look for use of accessory muscles and any audible sounds such as a wheeze or secretions. Look at the patient's colour and skin. While taking the pulse, note how the patient's skin feels. Is it hot and sweaty or cold and clammy? If you have a portable BP monitor, obtain the BP.

Q2. Reassure the patient and inform the case manager or community matron. You may wish to contact his GP and any family members. If you are unable to make contact with the medical or nursing staff, you may need to consider telephoning for an emergency ambulance. Try to optimise the patient's breathing by sitting him upright and minimising exertion.

Practice point 3.2

Q1. The most important observation to record is the respiratory rate, rhythm and depth.

Q2. Secondary observations will be BP, pulse, temperature, SpO_2 and peak flow.

Q3. On completing the observations and calculating the early warning score, reassure and keep the patient as calm as possible. Consider inserting a cannula and obtain blood if available and if there is any cause for concern, inform a senior member of staff.

CHAPTER 4

Practice point 4.1

Exercise, diet, sleep, stress, hereditary, age and disease.

Practice point 4.2 – Cardiovascular case study

Q1. Observations to record: respiration, temperature, pulse, BP, saturations, EWS, fluid balance, pain assessment. Document the observations and inform the nurse in charge.

Q2. Look at the patient's skin – if she has been on holiday, skin may be sunburnt, red and swollen, sweaty. Look for any breaks in the skin. Look at the breathing pattern, rate and rhythm – is it fast or slow? Listen to the patient and talk to her about how she is feeling currently. Listen for any noisy breathing. Feel the skin for any signs of dry, dehydrated skin or warm, sweaty skin. Relay your finding to the nurse in charge.

Practice point 4.3

Answer will vary depending on your hospital practice. Compare with the national guidelines from www.survivingsepsis.org

CHAPTER 5

Practice point 5.1

The nurse should look for the nurse in charge and inform them of what she has observed and listen to what instructions the registered nurse issues. The nurse may be asked to mark/outline the area that is red so that it can be monitored. The nurse can obtain a temperature reading and report it to the staff nurse as well as feel for a pulse. A fast pulse may be another clue to the patient having an infected wound site. The nurse can also perform CRT and inform the nurse in charge, who should inform the surgical doctors as soon as possible. The nurse can check with the patient to find out about any allergy to wound dressings, as this may be a reason why the skin is red. The nurse should listen to the patient and find out if the wound is painful and whether the patient feels hot or cold. This should be reported to the nurse in charge, who may be able to administer some analgesia.

Practice point 5.2

The nurse should look at her grandfather and observe to see if he has got sun burnt while gardening. She should listen to what he tells her and she can ask him if he has been drinking plenty on the hot day and ask him if he has been having a lot of headaches. If he is having a lot of headaches, it may be useful for the nurse to discuss with her grandfather the option of visiting the GP for more tests. If the headache is unexpected, but he is warm and dehydrated, he may feel better once he has had something to eat and drink.

The nurse can feel her grandfather's skin and assess if it is hot or cold. This will provide more clues as to why he is feeling unwell.

CHAPTER 6

Practice point 6.1

To calculate the MAP for a BP of 120/60

$$MAP = Diastolic + \frac{(systolic - diastolic)}{3}$$

$$60 + \frac{(120 - 60)}{3} = MAP \text{ is } 80$$

Practice point 6.2

Sodium (Na)	135–145 mmol/l
Potassium (K)	3.5–5 mmol/l
Bicarbonate (HCO₃)	22–30 mmol/l
Creatinine	35–125 μmol/l
Urea	<6.6 mmol/l

Practice point 6.3

Chart (1) is poorly documented. Although it tells you that some drinks were left, it does not say how much was drunk. Staff may be documenting these drinks on the drinks round, but they do not check on how much the input was. It tells you that the patient used the toilet but not how much the output was. To improve this, patients should be shown how to measure their drinks and be involved in the documentation. The patient also needs to know where the bed pans are such that the urine can be weighed or measured. Chart (2) is more accurate and also has a cumulative balance.

Practice point 6.4

Compare strengths and weaknesses of local fluid balance charts in relation to accuracy and information on fluid input and output.

Practice point 6.5a

To calculate Mr Walkers ideal urine output, multiple his body weight in kg by 0.5–1.0 ml per hour.

$$70 \times 0.5 = 35 \text{ ml}$$

$$70 \times 1.0 = 70 \text{ ml}$$

Therefore, the urine output should range between 35 ml and 70 ml per hour.

Practice point 6.5b

First action should be to inform the nurse in charge of the changes in the vital signs and the deterioration. Second, you can talk to Mr Walker and find out how he is currently feeling. His potential problems are that he is still dehydrated and is at risk of prerenal ARF. Mr Walker's catheter should also be checked to ensure that it is patent and is not blocked. He needs more fluids. If Mr Walker is no longer vomiting, he can be encouraged to drink more fluids orally. You can assist the nurse or doctor by ensuring that you have the equipment ready to assist them. You can also recheck the observations in 15 minutes and see if any of the actions have improved his BP, pulse and respiration. Record a track and trigger score.

CHAPTER 7

Practice point 7.1

Acute pain conditions	Chronic pain conditions
Acute pancreatitis	Spondylosis
Fractured ribs or bones	Rheumatoid arthritis
Post-operative wound pain	Back pains, arthritic hip or joints
Myocardial infarction	Migraines

These are a few examples and therefore not exclusive.

Practice point 7.2

Other factors to observe include the following:

Visual signs of pain such as grimacing, looking flushed, guarding the painful area and limited mobility. Reassure the patient and perform pain assessment at rest and at movement. Ask medical staff to prescribe analgesia with an anti-emetic (this is usually morphine and cyclizine). The fastest route for pain relief will be the IV route, although other routes may be chosen such as PR or IM. The patient will require oxygen therapy as saturations are low; recheck vital signs in 20–30 minutes and monitor effect of analgesia.

Practice point 7.3

Alfentanil	Step 3 analgesic for severe pain
Amitriptiline	Adjuvant medication
Aspirin	Step 1 analgesic for mild pain
Bupivocaine	Adjuvant medication
Carbamazipine	Adjuvant medication
Codeine	Step 2 analgesic for moderate pain
Dexamethsone	Adjuvant medication
Diamorphine	Step 3 analgesic for severe pain
Diazepam	Adjuvant medication
Fentanyl	Step 3 analgesic for severe pain

Gabapentin	Adjuvant medication
GTN spray	Adjuvant medication
Hydrocortisone	Adjuvant medication
Hydromorphone	Step 3 analgesic for severe pain
Ibrufen	Step 2 analgesic for moderate pain
Ketorolac	Step 3 analgesic for severe pain
Lignocaine	Adjuvant medication
Methadone	Step 3 analgesic for severe pain
Morphine	Step 3 analgesic for severe pain
MST	Step 3 analgesic for severe pain
Oromorph	Step 3 analgesic for severe pain
Oxycodone	Step 3 analgesic for severe pain
Paracetamol	Step 1 analgesic for mild pain
Pethidine	Step 3 analgesic for severe pain
Prednisolone	Adjuvant medication
Remifentanil	Step 3 analgesic for severe pain
Tramadol-	Step 2 analgesic for mild pain

CHAPTER 8

Practice point 8.1

Q1. The early warning score is 5.

Q2. You may also have noticed that the AVPU, EWS and MAP scores are not documented and not included.

Q3. The EWS has not triggered a correct score and the observation chart is incomplete.

Q4. It is also clear that a trend is appearing on the observation chart. The temperature, pulse and respiratory rate are raised and the blood pressure is going down.

Q5. The pigeon or seagull sign is also evident on the observations that were documented previously.

Q6. You need to follow the escalation policy with an EWS score of 5 and take action according to your scope of practice.

Practice point 8.2

Q1. Mrs Jones has an EWS of 6; if your practice area also includes a score for oxygen saturation and urine output, this also needs to be added to the total score.

Q2. It is clear that the clinical observations show that Mrs Jones is becoming acutely unwell and her consciousness level is deteriorating.

Q3. You need to follow the escalation policy with an EWS score of 5 and take action according to your scope of practice.

CHAPTER 9

Practice point 9.1

(a) Potential barriers include his loss of memory and change in his normal behaviour because of the infection. He could be more agitated and confused than usual. The severity of the Alzheimer's disease will impact on whether Mr Collins is able to talk and communicate verbally with nurses.

(b) Mrs Collins will be able to tell you specific changes to Mr Collins' behaviour. Mr Collins may be frightened of you if he has not met you before, so use of language and tone of voice will be important in encouraging Mr Collins to agree to have his observations done.

Practice point 9.2

This answer will be a personal reflection on methods on how consent was gained from the patient.

Practice point 9.3

Strategies and communication systems to deal with Mrs Peters include the following:

- EWS charts.
- Follow escalation policy for EWS using the graded response.
- Contact senior staff – for example, doctor or nurse in charge.

- Review prescription sheet to find out what analgesia Mrs Peters can have.
- Call the Acute Pain Team for support and advice.

CHAPTER 11

Practice point 11.1

Q1. Mrs Brown is becoming hypoglycaemic as her blood sugar is below 3 mmol. The clinical observations show an EWS of 5 and she is sweating and confused. The symptoms provide a clear indication that if she is not treated quickly, she may become unconscious.

Q2. Locate the hypoglycaemic box and provide a sugary drink depending on her consciousness level; alternatively, administer glucagon if prescribed or contact the doctor.
Follow the escalation policy as her EWS is 5.
Recheck the blood sugar level in 15 minutes and if blood sugar level remains low, provide another sugary drink.

Practice point 11.2

Q1. Once you have read the policy and guidelines within your clinical area, reflect on your practice to ensure that you are adhering to the trust policy and guidelines. If you are not sure how to calibrate the blood glucose monitor, contact the Education and Training department for a relevant training session or contact a specialist diabetic nurse.

Q2. As an employee, you have a responsibility not only to understand but also to adhere to your employer's policy and guidelines. It is also your responsibility to be able to understand and use the equipment competently.

CHAPTER 12

Practice point 12.1

Mrs Cameron was SOB this am and mobilised UTT between 2 nurses. ~~On returning to bed, pt~~ took H_2O and diet orally. Vital signs are satisfactory. All cares given. SN ERB

Errors – SOB could mean shortness of breath or sat out of bed. UTT is not a recognised abbreviation for up to toilet. If mistakes are made, a single line should be struck through the incorrect documentation and dated and signed. 'Vital signs are satisfactory' provides insufficient information about the patient's physiological status and does not tell the healthcare team whether these are normal or not. 'All cares given' is also lacking in detail.

The document is only signed with abbreviated signature, which does not include the date and time and designation of the staff. SN could be equated to student nurse or staff nurse. The signature should be recorded on the same line as the last piece of documentation or a single line drawn through to prevent any further tampering with the record. In a court of law, if this care plan was requested as evidence, there would be implications for the quality of care and the nursing recording the information.

The correct way to record the care plan

10/06/2010. 12.00 hrs. Documented retrospectively – Mrs Cameron was sat out of bed this morning and mobilised up to the toilet, supported by two nurses. Mrs Cameron was assisted by myself and the student nurse with washing and dressing. Patient cleaned her own teeth and brushed her own hair independently. Tissue viability checked and assessed as intact with no pressure sores. On returning to her chair, the patient had water and sugar-free diet orally. Vital signs were taken at 10 am. Temperature 37.2, respiratory rate 14, blood pressure 135/75, pulse 92 and regular

SN ERB   (Staff Nurse E.R. Butterworth, Band 5).

CHAPTER 14

Practice point 14.1

This answer will be a personal reflection on the methods on how to perform BP using the correct cuff size using Gibb's reflective cycle that involves the following:

Describe what happened.
Examine your thoughts, feelings and behaviour.
Examine the thoughts, feelings and behaviour of others involved.
Analyse the situation. How do you know?
Consider what other options were open to you.
Identify your actions if the situation arose again.

Practice point 14.2

The white hat – provides information	Ask Mr Leonard the reasons why he does not want his meal. Is it how the food has been presented? Is he feeling sick? Has he a sore mouth or faulty dentures? Does he require a special diet? Does he require assistance with eating?
The red hat – provides feelings and emotions	Ask Mr Leonard about how he is feeling and if there is any action that can improve his emotions and feelings. Is he feeling low or depressed? Is he lethargic because of the chemotherapy? Has he a sore mouth or mouth infection that is affecting his appetite?

Continued

The black hat – provides caution and asks for care Highlights weakness and risk	Maintain Mr Leonard's privacy and dignity. Refer to hospital policy regarding nutrition
	Perform a MUST assessment
	Consider contacting the dietician
	Commence a food diary to monitor Mr Leonard's intake. The risks to Mr Leonard are high as he is immunocompromised and requires nutrition to heal and prevent infection.
	Mr Leonard should be supported to make his own decisions with all the information relevant to him
The yellow hat – provides optimism and positivity Looks at the benefits	Mr Leonard needs to be encouraged to look at the potential benefits of the chemotherapy and the benefit of eating and drinking. Eating and drinking should assist in preventing mouth infections. Consider the benefits of eating from a social perspective
The green hat – provides creativity and new ideas, allows for growth and development	Ask Mr Leonard if he can suggest any solutions – does he want small, more frequent snacks? Does he want a nutritional drink? Would regular anti-emetics help?
The blue hat – provides control and organisation of thinking	Discuss with Mr Leonard the potential solutions and incorporate into his care plan and ensure that the multidisciplinary team is aware of his revised nutritional plan
	Ensure that MUST, Waterlow Scores, Falls Assessments are completed

CHAPTER 15
Answers to the multiple choice questions (MCQ)

Infection control
What is the body's first line of defence?
(b) Skin

How are micro-organisms spread?
(e) All of the above

How many levels are there in the chain of infection?
(c) 6

How many steps are there in the hand washing procedure?
(d) 7

How long should it take to wash your hands?

(c) 15–30 seconds

The cardiovascular system
The blood leaves the heart at the
(b) left ventricle

Name the three layers of the heart.
(a) Endocardium
(b) Pericardium
(c) Myocardium

The blood pressure consists of

(d) all of the above

The normal pulse rate is

(b) 60–100 bpm

Respiratory
The respiratory systems consists of
(e) all of the above

The normal respiratory rate is

(b) 12–20 bpm

When we breathe out it is called
(c) expiration

The breathing patterns are

(d) all of the above

The most sensitive indicator that the patient is becoming unwell is
(c) the respirations

Early warning score
What score triggers a response?
(c) 3

What does AVPU mean?

(c) Conscious level

The pulse above the systolic blood pressure is called
(b) pigeon sign
(c) seagull sign

What causes an inaccurate reading on a pulse oximeter?
(e) All of the above

Continued

Pain

The meninges are

(d) all of the above

The body produces natural analgesics called
(b) endorphins
(d) encephalin

Record keeping

Written documentation should be recorded in
(c) black

Documentation needs to be

(e) all of the above

Nutrition

Which tool assesses nutritional status?
(e) MUST tool

How much water does the body need daily?
(a) 1–2 l
(b) 2–4 l
(c) 4–5 l
(d) 2–3 l

A normal BMI is

(d) 19–25

Communication

What are the barriers to communication?
(e) All of the above

An acronym for communication is
(a) SOLER
(b) SBAR

Diabetes

The normal level for blood sugar is
(c) 4–7 mmol

If the blood sugar is low the condition is called
(b) hypoglycaemia

Urine

The kidneys

(e) all of the above

How do we calculate urine output?
(b) Patients weight

The hormones produced by the kidneys are
(a) renin
(b) vitamin D
(c) erythropoietin
(d) prostaglandins

(*continued*)

Continued

The best route for nutrition is

(c) oral

Legal and ethical
Unqualified healthcare staff
are
(a) responsible
(b) accountable
What are the ethical
principles?
(e) All of the above

Valid consent is

(d) All of the above

Professional development
Developing your knowledge
and skills is a key element in
(e) all of the above

How much blood from the
heart do the kidney's need to
produce urine?
(c) 25%

Temperature
Where do we measure the
temperature?
(e) All of the above

A normal temperature is

(a) 36.8

The amount of insensible loss
is
(d) 500 ml

Reflection
A model of reflection is

(e) all of the above

Index

Vital Signs for Nurses: An Introduction to Clinical Observations, First Edition.
Joyce Smith and Rachel Roberts.
© 2011 Joyce Smith and Rachel Roberts. Published 2011 by Blackwell Publishing Ltd.